MITRAL VALVE PROLAPSE

Collected Reprints
(1985-2014)

By

WILLIAM C. ROBERTS, MD

and

COLLEAGUES

ISBN: 979-8-88862-161-5
Printed in the United States of America on acid-free paper.

Preface

In the beginning, mitral valve prolapse was an auscultatory finding with either a late or holosystolic precordial murmur. Then, its angiographic features were described via left ventricular angiogram. Then, its echocardiographic features were described, and lastly, its morphologic features. The collections included herein stress its morphologic features, particularly #1619, which illustrates these features.

—William C. Roberts, MD

Table of Contents

*Articles are numbered based on WCR's CV.

Mitral Valve Prolapse and Systemic Hypertension

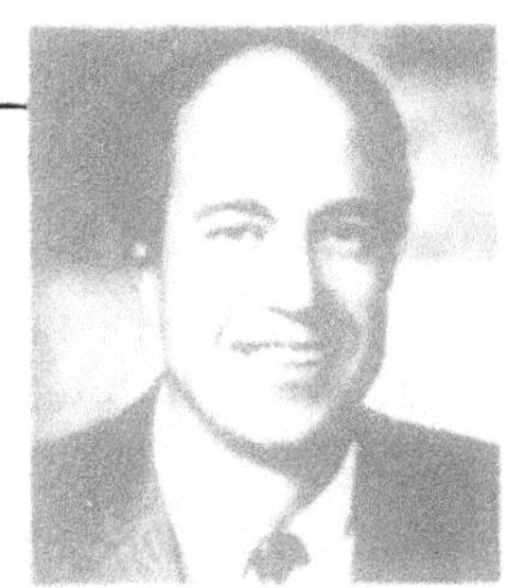

In the USA there are approximately 160 million persons over 20 years of age (total population = 238 million). Of the 160 million, an estimated 8 million (5%) have auscultatory evidence of mitral valve prolapse (MVP) and 60 million (37%) have systemic hypertension (SH) (arterial pressure $\geq$ 140/90 mm Hg). Accordingly, of the 8 million with MVP, nearly 3 million (0.37 $\times$ 8) have SH, and of the 60 million with SH, 3 million (0.05 $\times$ 60) have MVP. The number of persons, therefore, with both MVP and SH in the USA is substantial.

Except in the person with left ventricular outflow obstruction, the systemic peak systolic arterial pressure is identical to the left ventricular peak systolic pressure, which of course is the pressure that closes the mitral valve orifice during ventricular systole. The normal mitral valve withstands elevation of the left ventricular peak systolic pressure without development of mitral regurgitation unless mitral anular calcific deposition is heavy, a process which is more frequent in hypertensive than in normotensive persons.[1] But how well does the defective, i.e., prolapsed or floppy, mitral valve tolerate chronic elevation of the left ventricular peak systolic pressure? My answer is "poorly," and the reason is because the associated SH (specifically, the elevated left ventricular systolic pressure) greatly increases the frequency of spontaneous rupture of mitral chordae tendineae, an occurrence virtually limited to patients with preexisting MVP. Jeresaty and associates[2] found underlying MVP in 23 (92%) of 25 patients with spontaneous rupture of mitral chordae tendineae and Hickey and associates[3] found underlying MVP in 29 (94%) of 31 patients with spontaneous rupture of mitral chordae tendineae. In an earlier study,[4] my colleagues and I examined 60 operatively excised purely regurgitant prolapsed mitral valves: 13 had ruptured chordae tendineae and of these, 11 (85%) had had SH before valve replacement; of the remaining 47 valves, none had ruptured chordae tendineae and only 11 (23%) of them had had SH preoperatively.

The normal mitral leaflets, as with the leaflets of all 4 cardiac valves, consist of 2 components: the fibrosa and the spongiosa. The fibrosa consists of collagen fibrils and the spongiosa, of an acid mucopolysaccharide material. In MVP the collagen fibrils of both the leaflets and chordae tendineae are defective[5] and probably, at least initially, decreased in number, and the spongiosa material, the "weaker" of the 2 components, is present in excessive amounts. It is reasonable to believe that the weaker the mitral leaflet and chordal structures, the greater the effect on them of the left ventricular systolic pressure, and the greater the mitral closing pressure the greater its effect on the defective mitral leaflet and chordal structures.

In summary, the normal mitral valve tolerates elevated left ventricular systolic pressures (mitral closing pressures) well, i.e., without creating mitral regurgitation and without rupturing mitral chordae tendineae. The prolapsed mitral valve, in contrast, contains defective collagen fibrils and excess spongiosa and it appears to withstand elevated left ventricular systolic pressures poorly as manifested by a high frequency of spontaneous rupture of chordae tendineae (and probably also by an increased degree of leaflet prolapse). Thus, proper treatment of SH may prevent or delay the appearance of severe mitral regurgitation that occurs in some patients with MVP.

William C. Roberts, MD
Editor in Chief

1. **Roberts WC.** Morphologic features of the normal and abnormal mitral valve. Am J Cardiol 1983;51:1005–1028.
2. **Jeresaty RM, Edwards JE, Chawla SK.** Mitral valve prolapse and ruptured chordae tendineae. Am J Cardiol 1985;55:138–142.
3. **Hickey AJ, Wilcken DEL, Wright JS, Warren BA.** Primary (spontaneous) chordal rupture: relation to myxomatous valve disease and mitral valve prolapse. JACC 1985;5:1341–1346.
4. **Waller BF, Morrow AG, Maron BJ, Del Negro AA, Kent KM, McGrath FJ, Wallace RB, McIntosh CL, Roberts WC.** Etiology of clinically isolated, severe, chronic, pure mitral regurgitation: an analysis of 97 patients over 30 years of age having mitral valve replacement. Am Heart J 1982;104:276–288.
5. **Renteria VG, Ferrans VJ, Jones M, Roberts WC.** Intracellular collagen fibrils in prolapsed ("floppy") human atrioventricular valves. Lab Invest 1976;35:439–443.

Mechanisms of severe mitral regurgitation in mitral valve prolapse determined from analysis of operatively excised valves

Certain clinical and mitral valvular morphologic findings are described in 83 patients (age 26 to 79 years [mean, 60]; 26 women [31%] and 57 men [69%]) with mitral valve prolapse (MVP) and mitral regurgitation (MR) severe enough to warrant mitral valve replacement. All 83 operatively excised valves were examined by the same person, and all excised valves had been purely regurgitant (no element of stenosis). No patients had hemodynamic evidence of dysfunction of the aortic valve. In each valve a portion of the posterior mitral leaflet was elongated such that the distance from the distal margin to basal attachment of this leaflet was similar to the distance from the distal margin of the anterior leaflet to its basal attachment to the left atrial wall. Two major mechanisms for the severe MR were found: (1) dilatation of the mitral anulus with or without rupture of chordae tendineae and (2) rupture of chordae tendineae with or without dilatation of the mitral anulus. Of the 83 patients, 48 (58%) had both dilated anuli (>11 cm in circumference) and ruptured chordae tendineae; 16 (19%) had dilated anuli without ruptured chordae, and 16 (19%) had ruptured chordae without significant anular dilatation. In three patients the anulus was not dilated, nor were chordae ruptured, and therefore the mechanism of the MR is uncertain. Mitral chordal rupture was nearly as frequent in the 64 patients with clearly dilated anular circumferences as in the 19 patients with normal or insignificantly dilated anular circumferences (≤11 cm). (AM HEART J 1987;113:1316.)

William C. Roberts, M.D., Charles L. McIntosh, M.D., Robert B. Wallace, M.D.,
Bethesda, Md. and Washington, D.C.

Mitral valve prolapse (MVP) is recognized to occur clinically in about 5% of persons over 20 years of age. In the United States, approximately 160 million persons are over 20 years of age, 8 million of whom have MVP. In most persons with clinical evidence of MVP, no symptoms are produced by the prolapsed valve. Although many persons with MVP have auscultatory evidence of minimal or mild mitral regurgitation (MR), the development of severe MR, severe enough to require operative intervention, is uncommon. This article describes certain findings in 83 patients who had MVP and MR severe enough to warrant mitral valve replacement.

PATIENTS STUDIED

The surgical pathology files of the Pathology Branch, National Heart, Lung, and Blood Institute, were searched for persons who had had mitral valve excision for pure MR. All valves had been so classified initially by W.C.R. Nearly 300 cases were so classified. Many cases were eliminated because either the operatively excised valve was no longer available or photographs of the operatively excised valve were unavailable. Some cases were eliminated because it was apparent that the cause of the pure MR was the following: (1) *rheumatic heart disease* (diffuse fibrosis of both mitral leaflets without elongation of the basal to distal margin of the posterior leaflet), (2) *infective endocarditis* involving a previously normal valve or one previously affected by rheumatic heart disease, (3) *papillary muscle dysfunction* from coronary artery disease (necrotic or fibrotic papillary muscle in the absence of either significant mitral anular dilatation or posterior mitral leaflet elongation), (4) *hypertrophic cardiomyopathy* or (5) *systemic lupus erythematosus* or *hypereosinophilic syndrome*. Some cases were eliminated because the aortic valve had also been excised simultaneously or because the aortic valve was found to have functioned abnormally: either stenotic or regurgitant or both. A few cases were eliminated because on review of preoperative hemody-

From the Pathology and Surgery Branches, National Heart, Lung, and Blood Institute, National Institutes of Health, and the Department of Surgery, Georgetown University.

Reprint requests: William C. Roberts, M.D., Pathology Branch, Bldg. 10A, Room 3E-30, National Heart, Lung, and Blood Institute, National Institutes of Health, Bethesda, MD 20892.

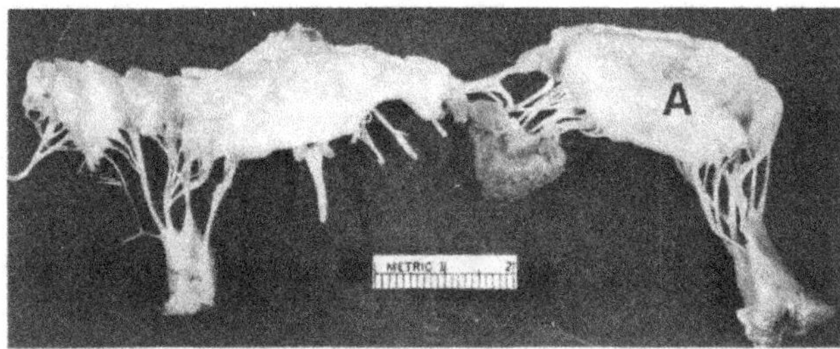

Fig. 1. Operatively excised mitral valve in a 56-year-old man (S68-4175). The anular circumference measures about 11 cm. Some chordae tendineae from the posterior leaflet are missing. The distance from site of attachment (anulus) to distal margin of both posterior and anterior *(A)* leaflets is similar. The atrial surface of the leaflets is shown.

namic data a small mean diastolic gradient had been recorded between the left atrium or pulmonary arterial wedge position and the left ventricle, and therefore the patient did not have "pure" MR.

A total of 83 cases were collected in which preoperative cardiac catheterization had indicated that the hemodynamic lesion involving the mitral valve was *pure* regurgitation, that the aortic valve had functioned normally (no element of either stenosis or regurgitation), and that examination of the operatively excised mitral valve had indicated that it fulfilled the following morphologic definition of MVP: in a portion of the posterior mitral leaflet the distance from its distal margin to its attachment at the mitral anulus was clearly elongated, a finding not observed in patients in whom the MR resulted from other causes, namely, rheumatic, infective endocarditis, coronary artery disease, hypertrophic cardiomyopathy, systemic lupus erythematosus, or hypereosinophilic syndrome. Usually at some point the distance from basal attachment to distal margin of the posterior mitral leaflet was similar to the distance from the distal margin of the anterior mitral leaflet to the point where the left atrial wall contacted it. The elongation of the posterior mitral leaflet caused an increase in the area of this leaflet. Many patients also had dilated mitral anuli, and the chordae in many patients appeared to be longer than usual. This latter finding, however, could not be systematically evaluated because many of the operatively excised mitral valves did not include attached papillary muscles. Photographs of the operatively excised mitral valves were available in 81 (98%) of the 83 patients. Of the 83 cases, 42 (51%) had been included in a previous publication concerning the various causes of pure MR severe enough to warrant mitral valve replacement.[1] More-

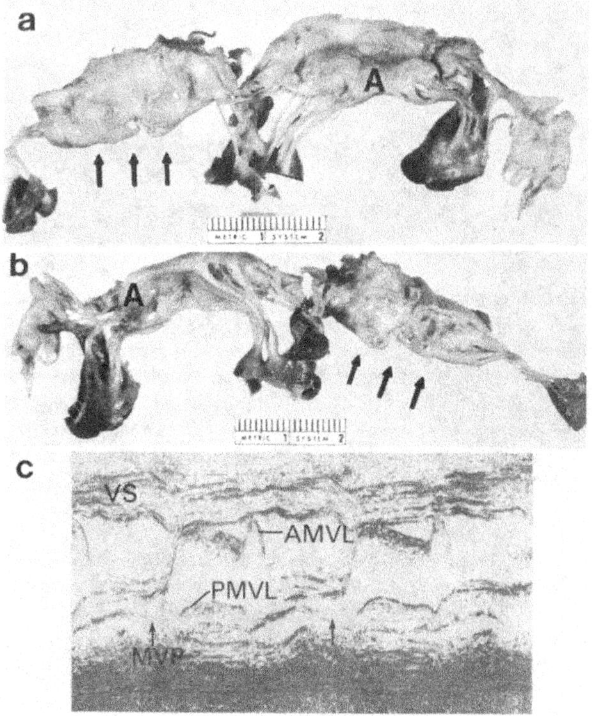

Fig. 2. Operatively excised mitral valve *(a* and *b)* and echocardiogram *(c)* recorded 1 month before valve replacement in a 43-year-old man (S70-3086). *a,* Atrial surface; *b,* Ventricular surface. Chordae are missing from the posterior leaflet *(arrows).* The distance from the site of attachment to distal margin of both anterior *(A)* and posterior leaflets is similar. *c,* The echocardiogram shows prolapse of the posterior leaflet. AMVL = anterior mitral valve leaflet; PMVL = posterior mitral valve leaflet; VS = ventricular septum.

over, 25 (30%) of the 83 cases had been included in a previous publication concerning the frequency of calcific deposits in mitral valves excised because of pure MR.[2]

The operation to replace the mitral valve in the 83 patients had been performed at four different medical centers, and the operatively excised valve in each was thereafter submitted to the Pathology Branch of the National Heart, Lung, and Blood Institute for examination. The valve was weighed, its anular circumference was measured, and a determination was made whether chordae tendineae attached to both leaflets were "disrupted" or "missing" or neither. Chordae were considered "disrupted" if detached chordae had rounded or blunted distal ends that were thicker than normal, often thicker than the more proximal portions of the same chordae. Chordae were considered "missing" if none extended caudally beneath the ventricular surfaces of a portion of either or both leaflets. Both "dis-

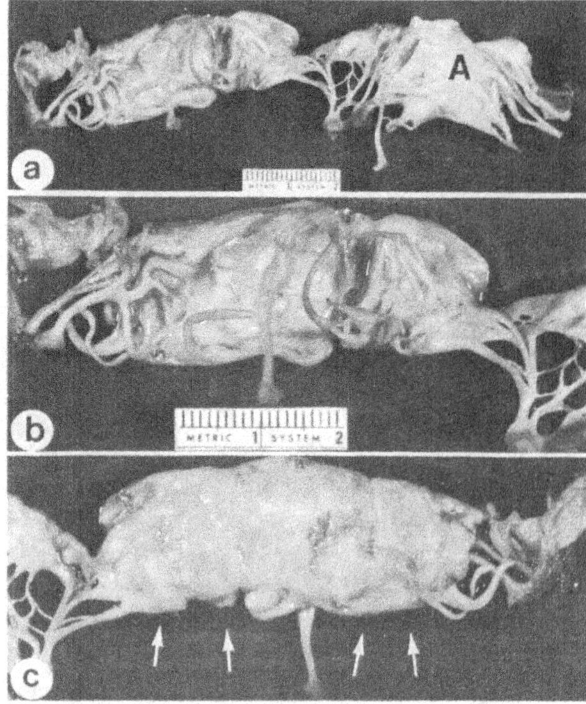

Fig. 3. Operatively excised mitral valve in a 55-year-old woman (S76-35). The anulus measures about 12 cm in circumference. Most chordae from the posterior leaflet are missing *(arrows)*. a, Ventricular aspect of valve. b, Ventricular aspect of posterior leaflet. c, Atrial aspect of posterior leaflet.

rupted" and "missing" chordae were considered "ruptured" chordae.

RESULTS

The 83 patients included 26 women (31%) and 57 men (69%). The women at the time of mitral valve replacement ranged in age from 42 to 79 years (mean, 61 years) and the men ranged from 26 to 77 years (mean, 59 years). The 26-year-old man had the Marfan syndrome. The next youngest patient was 42 years old. Of the 83 patients, 15 (18%) were younger than 51 years old, and 68 patients (82%) were older than 50 years of age at the time of mitral valve replacement. The excised valves (Figs. 1 to 18) ranged in weight from 4.0 to 14.5 gm (mean, 6.7 gm). The larger weights were in the valves in which one or both papillary muscles had usually been excised. Calcific deposits were present in 28 valves (34%). The calcific deposits involved primarily the mitral anular region in 19 patients (68%), one or both mitral leaflets without anular involvement in three patients (11%), one or more chordae tendineae only in four patients (14%), and papillary muscle only in two patients (7%). The calcific deposits were focal and small in all patients.

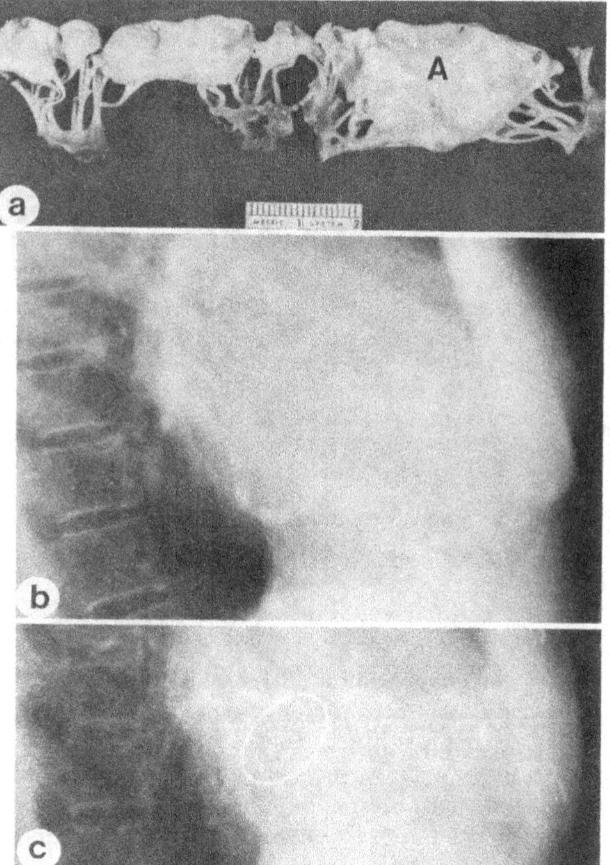

Fig. 4. Operatively excised mitral valve *(a)* showing its atrial aspect and lateral radiographs showing a C-shaped calcific deposit before *(b)* and after *(c)* valve replacement in a 47-year-old woman (S76-156). Some chordae from the posterior leaflet are missing. A = anterior leaflet.

The circumference of the mitral anulus in the 26 women ranged from 9 to 15 cm (mean, 12). It was ≤11 cm in 10 patients (38%), and nine (90%) had missing or disrupted chordae tendineae. The circumference was >11 cm in 16 women (62%), and 13 (81%) had missing or disrupted chordae. Of the 26 women, 22 (85%) had ruptured chordae. In the 57 men, the mitral anular circumference ranged from 10 to 18 cm (mean, 14). It was ≤11 cm in nine patients (16%), and seven of the nine had missing or disrupted chordae. It was >11 cm in 48 men (84%), and 35 (73%) had missing or disrupted chordae. Of the 57 men, 42 (74%) had ruptured chordae. Of the entire 83 patients, 64 (77%) had missing or disrupted chordae: in 16 (84%) of the 19 patients in whom the anular circumference was ≤11 cm and in 48 (75%) of the 64 in whom the anular circumference was >11 cm.

Of the 64 (77%) patients with missing or disrupted chordae or both, the missing or disrupted

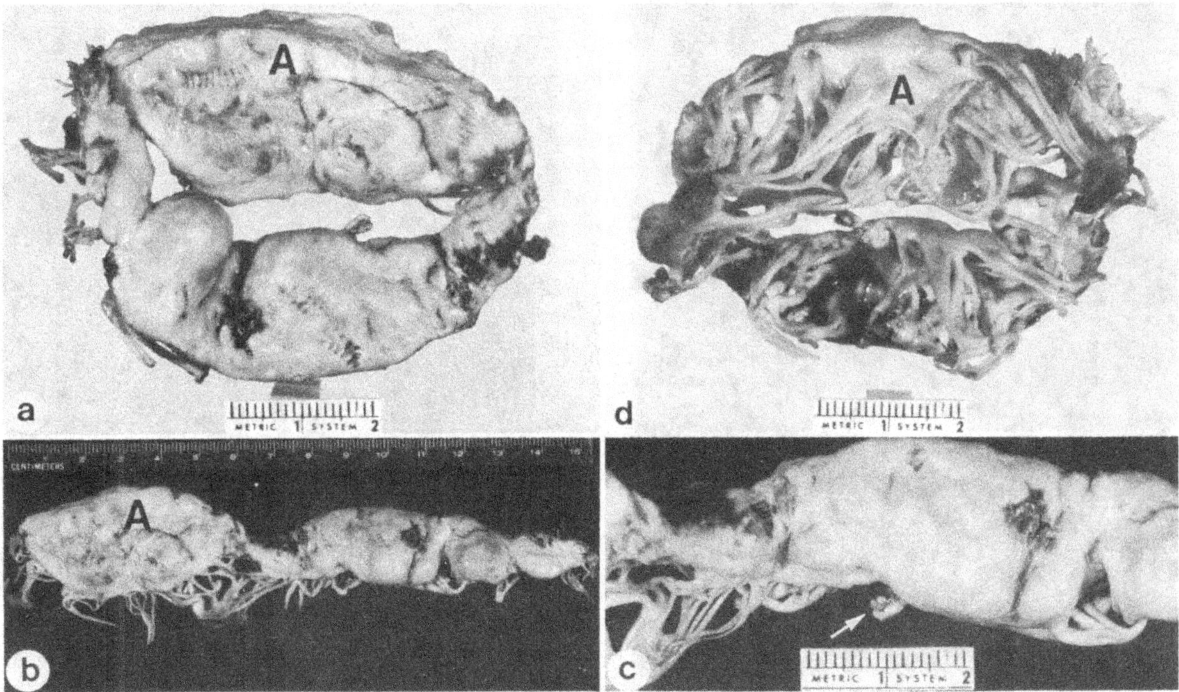

Fig. 5. Operatively excised mitral valve in a 60-year-old man (S77-157). *a-c* Atrial aspect. *d*, Ventricular aspect. Both anterior *(A)* and posterior leaflets are of similar size. Chordae from the posterior leaflet are both missing and disrupted. The disrupted chord is designated by the arrow. *c*, A close-up of the posterior leaflet. (Reproduced with permission from Byram MT and Roberts WC. Frequencies and extent of calcific deposits in purely regurgitant mitral valves: analysis of 108 operatively excised valves. Am J Cardiol 1983;52:1059-61.)

chordae involved the posterior leaflet only in 57 patients (90%), the anterior leaflet only in three patients (5%), and both leaflets in three patients (5%). In all 57 patients in whom only chordae to the posterior leaflet were affected, the chordae were considered missing in each. In the three patients in whom only chordae to the anterior leaflet were affected, the chordae were considered disrupted in one, missing in one, and both disrupted and missing in one. Finally in the three patients in whom chordae from both leaflets were affected, in each some chordae were disrupted and some were missing. No patient with missing chordae had historical evidence of infective endocarditis that had healed, and therefore the chordal rupture in them is considered "spontaneous." Of the eight patients with disrupted chordae with or without missing chordae, five had historical evidence of infective endocarditis that had healed.

DISCUSSION

The above data indicate that there are two major mechanisms for development of severe MR in MVP: (1) dilatation of the mitral anulus with or without rupture of chordae tendineae and (2) rupture of chordae tendineae with or without dilatation of the mitral anulus. Of our 83 patients with MVP, severe MR, and mitral valve replacement, 48 (58%) had both dilated anuli (>11 cm in circumference) and ruptured chordae tendineae; 16 (19%) had dilated anuli without rupture of chordae, and 16 (19%) had ruptured chordae without significant anular dilatation. In three of the 83 patients, the anulus was not dilated, nor were chordae ruptured. Therefore the mechanism of the severe MR in these three patients is unclear. Mitral chordal rupture was nearly as frequent in the 64 patients with clearly dilated mitral anuli (circumference >11 cm) as in the 19 patients with normal or insignificantly dilated anuli (circumference ≤11 cm) (75% [48/64] vs 84% [16/19]).

The reported frequencies of rupture of chordae tendineae in operatively excised prolapsed (floppy) mitral valves have not been as high as in the present study. The explanation almost surely lies in differing definitions of the term "ruptured chordae tendineae." In the present study only nine patients (11%) had easily identifiable, unequivocally disrupted

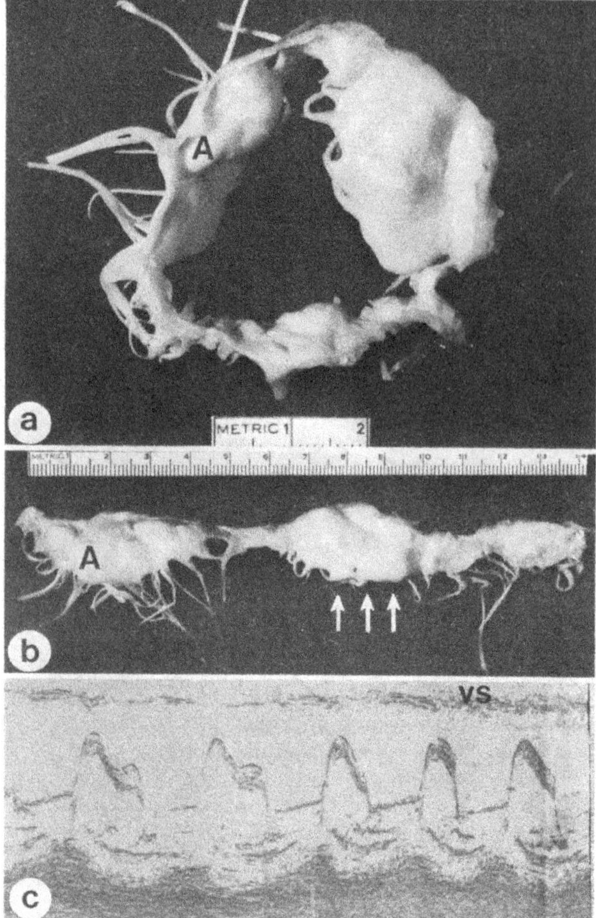

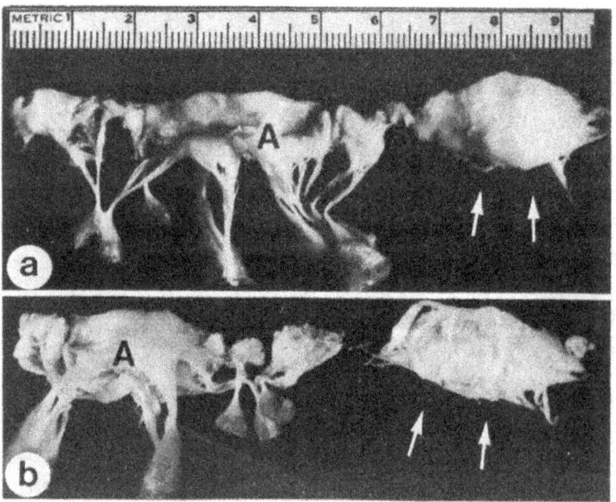

Fig. 6. Operatively excised mitral valve (*a* and *b*) and preoperative echocardiogram (*c*) in a 64-year-old man (S80-64). The anulus is nearly 15 cm in circumference. Chordae from the posterior leaflet are missing *(arrows). c,* Echocardiogram showing prolapse *(arrows).* A = anterior leaflet; VS = ventricular septum.

Fig. 7. Atrial *(a)* and ventricular *(b)* aspects of the excised mitral valve in a 70-year-old woman (S80-162). The anulus is only about 10 cm in circumference. Many chordae from the posterior leaflet are missing *(arrows).*

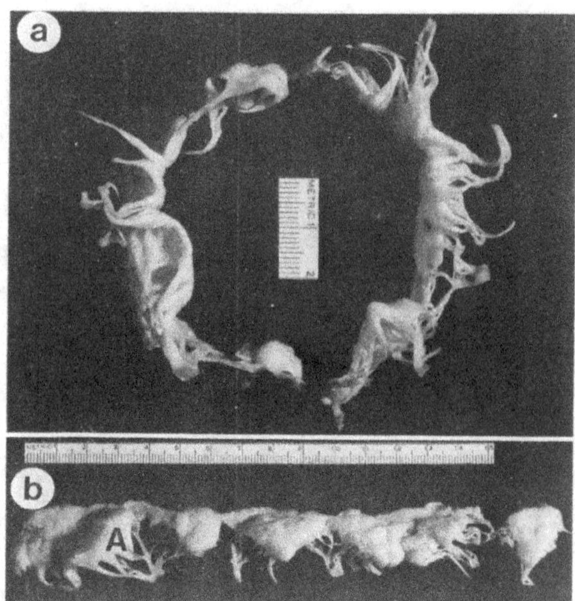

Fig. 8. Intact *(a)* and opened *(b)* operatively excised mitral valve in a 67-year-old man (S80-172). The anulus is enormously dilated (17 cm). Some chordae from the posterior leaflet are missing. A = anterior leaflet.

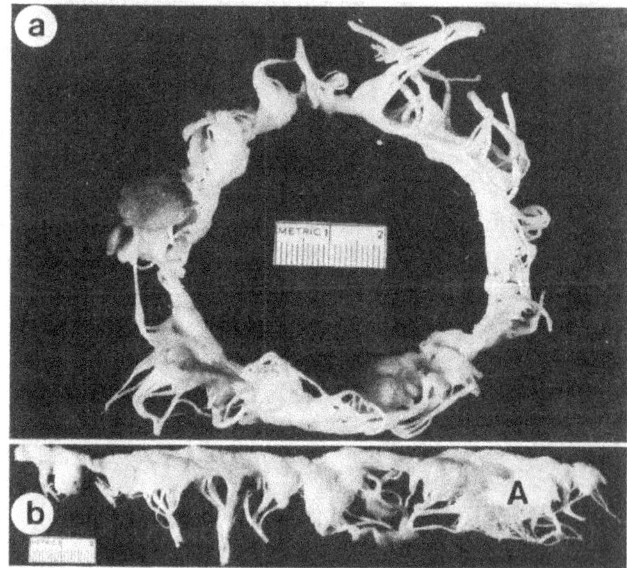

Fig. 9. Intact *(a)* and opened *(b)* operatively excised valve in a 26-year-old man (S82-1) who had the Marfan syndrome. This patient was the youngest in this study. The anulus is enormously dilated (about 18 cm). The chordae appear to be intact. A = anterior leaflet.

chordae. In contrast, 61 (73%) had no identifiable disrupted chordae, but portions of the posterior leaflet were devoid of chordae. These patients were considered to have "missing" chordae, a situation equivalent to disrupted chordae. Of the nine patients with disrupted chordae, seven also had

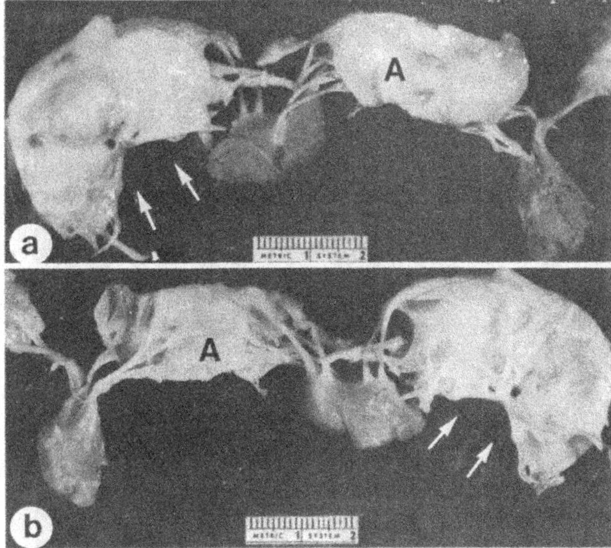

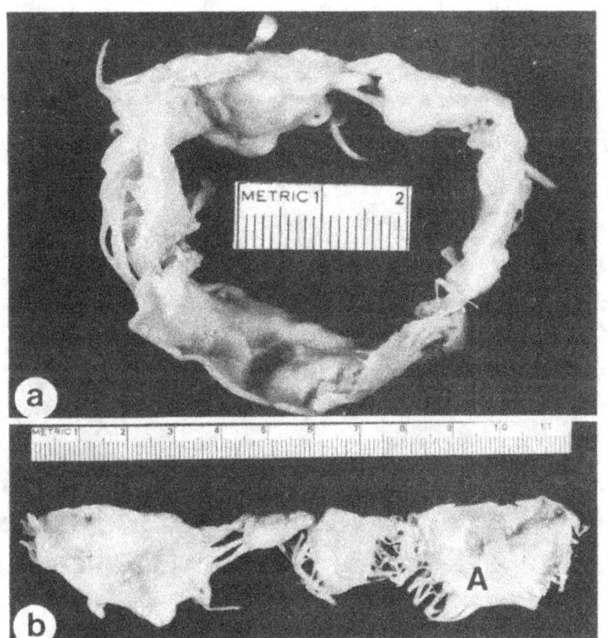

Fig. 10. Opened mitral valve showing the atrial *(a)* and ventricular *(b)* aspects in a 42-year-old woman (77S-3497). Both anterior *(A)* and posterior leaflets are of similar size. Many chordae from the posterior leaflet are missing. The anulus is about 13 cm in circumference.

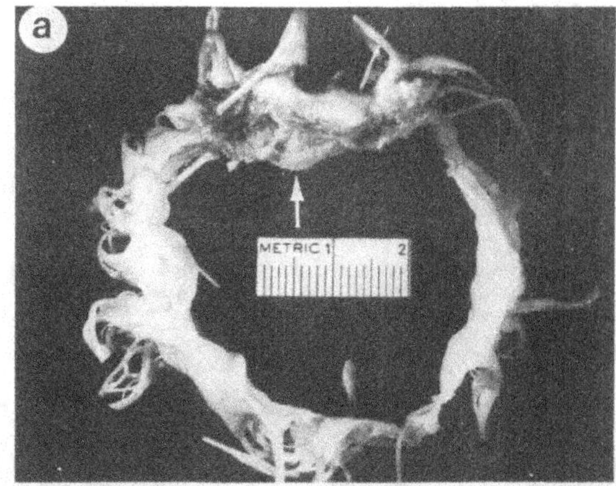

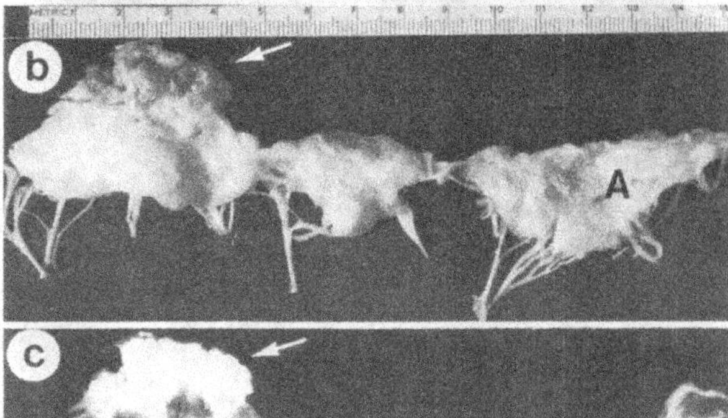

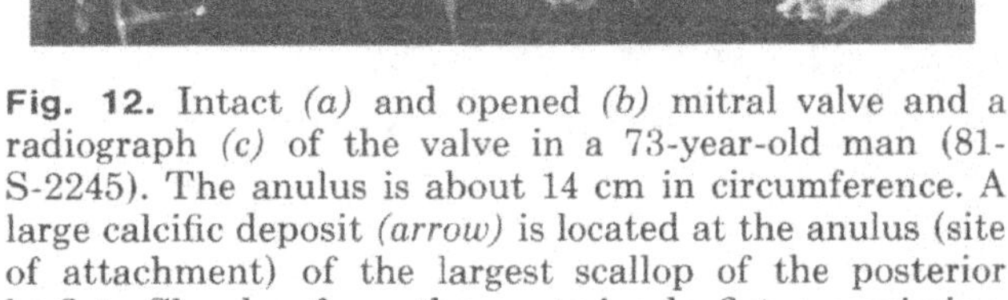

Fig. 11. Intact *(a)* and opened *(b)* mitral valve in a 65-year-old man (80-S-3326). The anulus is about 12 cm in circumference. Most chordae from the posterior leaflet are missing. A = anterior leaflet.

Fig. 12. Intact *(a)* and opened *(b)* mitral valve and a radiograph *(c)* of the valve in a 73-year-old man (81-S-2245). The anulus is about 14 cm in circumference. A large calcific deposit *(arrow)* is located at the anulus (site of attachment) of the largest scallop of the posterior leaflet. Chordae from the posterior leaflet are missing. A = anterior leaflet.

missing chordae. Of the 61 patients with missing chordae, seven also had disrupted chordae. Thus, only two of the 83 patients had disrupted without missing chordae.

The cause of the chordal rupture was not determined in 59 (92%) of the 64 patients, and therefore their chordal rupture is considered "spontaneous." It is now recognized that spontaneous rupture of mitral chordae tendineae is nearly always in the setting of MVP.[3-7] Of the 83 patients studied, at least six had a history of active infective endocarditis that had healed: five had disrupted mitral chordae and one had no disrupted or missing chordae. None of the 54 patients with missing but without disrupted chordae had had a history of active infective endocarditis.

Although MVP appears to be more common in women than in men, severe MR caused by MVP is more common in men. Of our 83 patients with MVR and MR severe enough to warrant mitral replacement, nearly 70% were men. In 23 patients with MVP and MR severe enough to warrant mitral valve replacement and reported by Jeresaty et al.,[3] at least 13 and probably 15 (65%) were men. Of 18 patients

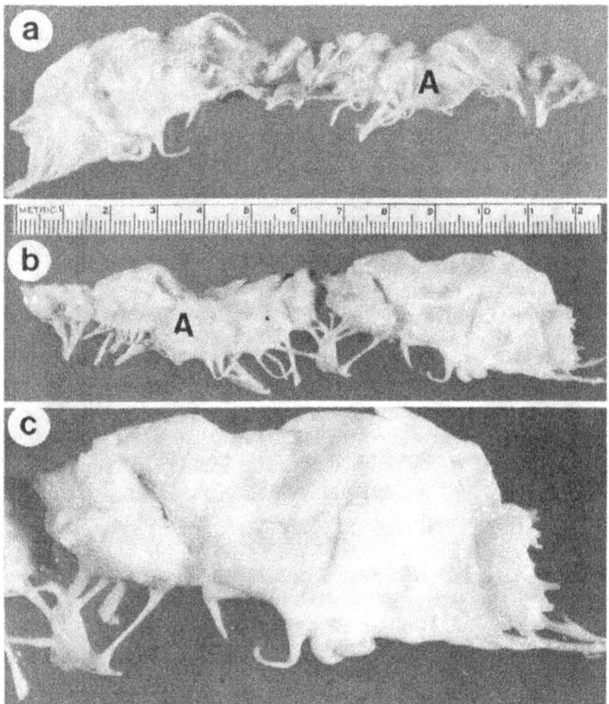

Fig. 13. Opened mitral valve (*a* and *b*) and close-up of portion of posterior leaflet *(c)* in a 58-year-old woman (83-S-3077). *a,* Ventricular aspect. *b,* Atrial aspect. *c,* Atrial aspect. The anulus is about 14 cm in circumference. Many chordae from the posterior leaflet are missing. A = anterior leaflet.

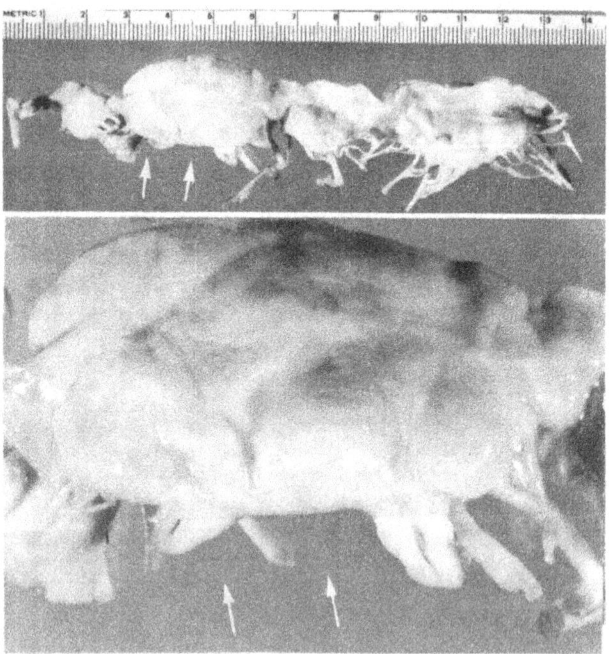

Fig. 14. Opened mitral valve from the atrial aspect in a 64-year-old woman (84-S-325). The anulus is nearly 14 cm in circumference. Many chordae from the posterior leaflet are missing *(arrows)*. A close-up of a portion of posterior leaflet is shown in the lower panel.

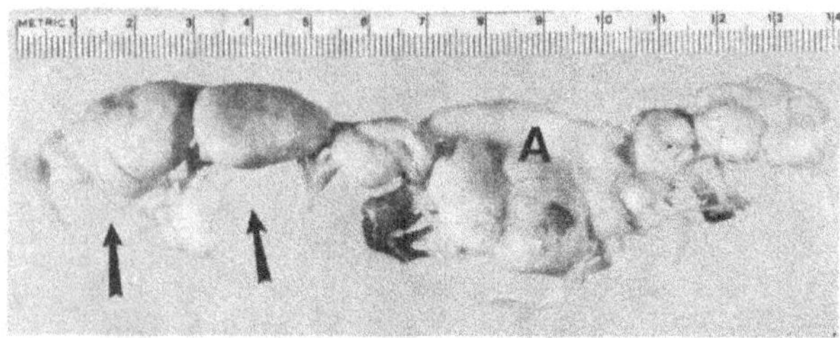

Fig. 15. Opened mitral valve showing its atrial aspects in a 65-year-old woman (84-S-3509). Many chordae from the posterior leaflet are missing *(arrows)*. The anulus is about 14 cm in circumference. A = anterior leaflet.

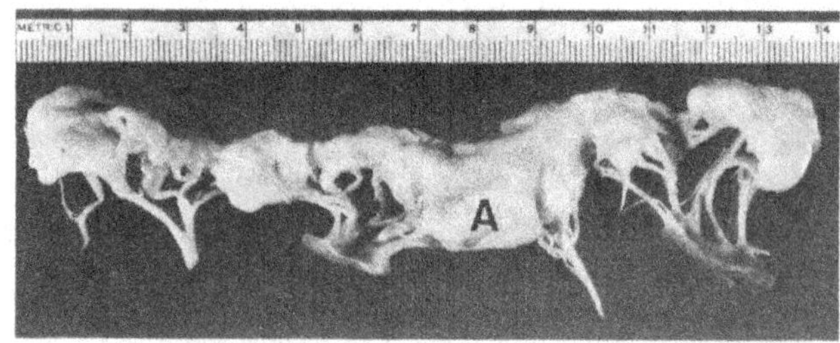

Fig. 16. Opened mitral valve showing its atrial aspect in a 71-year-old woman (84-S-7903). The anulus is about 14 cm in circumference. The chordae appear to be intact. A = anterior leaflet.

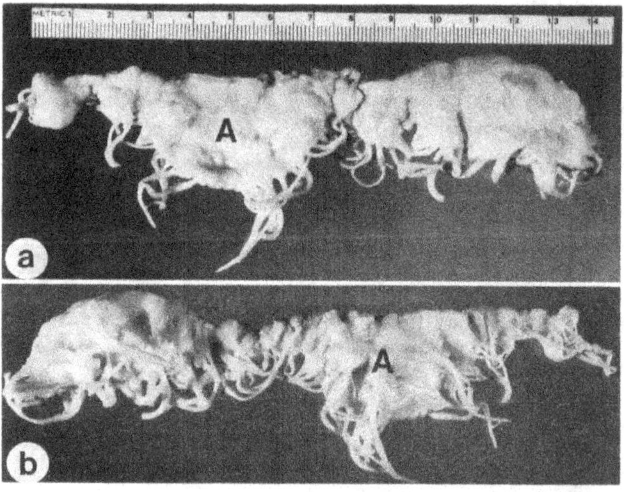

Fig. 17. Opened mitral valve showing its atrial *(a)* and ventricular *(b)* aspects in a 44-year-old man (85-S-971). The anulus is about 15 cm in circumference. Chordae from the posterior leaflet appear to be both missing and others disrupted. A = anterior leaflet.

with MVP and MR severe enough to warrant mitral replacement and reported by Olson et al.,[7] 14 (78%) were men. Of 11 patients ≥60 years of age with MVP and MR severe enough to warrant mitral replacement and reported by Naggar et al.,[8] six (55%) were men.

Finally, opportunities to study systematically

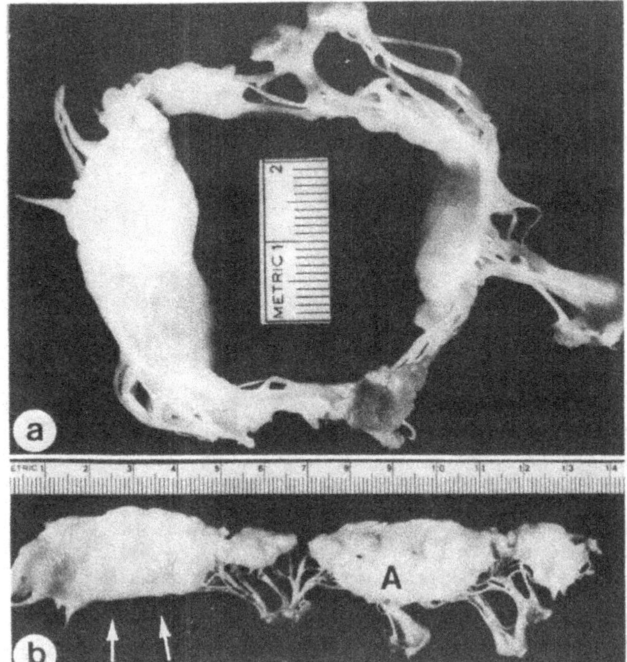

Fig. 18. Unopened *(a)* and opened *(b)* mitral valve in a 66-year-old man (85-S-2575). The anulus is about 14 cm in circumference. Many chordae from the posterior leaflet are missing *(arrows)*. A = anterior leaflet.

operatively excised prolapsed mitral valves in the future will almost surely diminish because of a move away from replacement in favor of repair procedures for patients with severe MR caused by MVP. Thus

the data collected in the present study will not likely be collected again in a relatively short period of time.

REFERENCES

1. Waller BF, Morrow AG, Maron BJ, Del Negro AA, Kent KM, McGrath FJ, Wallace RB, McIntosh CL, Roberts WC. Etiology of clinically isolated, severe, chronic, pure mitral regurgitation: Analysis of 97 patients over 30 years of age having mitral valve replacement. AM HEART J 1982;104:276-88.
2. Byram MT, Roberts WC. Frequency and extent of calcific deposits in purely regurgitant mitral valves: analysis of 108 operatively excised valves. Am J Cardiol 1983;52:1059-61.
3. Jeresaty RM, Edwards JE, Chawla SK. Mitral valve prolapse and ruptured chordae tendineae. Am J Cardiol 1985;55:138-42.
4. Hickey AJ, Wicker Del, Wright JS, Warren BA. Primary (spontaneous) chordal rupture: relation to myxomatous valve disease and mitral valve prolapse. J Am Coll Cardiol 1985;5:1341-6.
5. Roberts WC. Mitral valve prolapse and systemic hypertension. Am J Cardiol 1985;56:703.
6. Aronson RJ, Hoffman M, Algueti-Margulis A, Yust I. Spontaneous rupture of mitral chordae tendineae in hypertension. Am J Cardiol (In press, 1987)
7. Olson LJ, Subramanian R, Ackerman DM, Orszulak TA, Edwards WD. Surgical pathology of the mitral valve: a study of 712 cases spanning 21 years. Mayo Clin Proc 1987;62:22-34.
8. Naggar CZ, Pearson WN, Seljan MP. Frequency of complications of mitral valve prolapse in subjects aged 60 years and older. Am J Cardiol 1986;58:1209-12.

Morphologic Comparison of Patients With Mitral Valve Prolapse Who Died Suddenly With Patients Who Died From Severe Valvular Dysfunction or Other Conditions

ALLEN L. DOLLAR, MD,* WILLIAM C. ROBERTS, MD. FACC

Bethesda, Maryland

Clinical and necropsy findings are described in 56 patients with mitral valve prolapse: 15 patients, aged 16 to 69 years (mean 39), died suddenly and mitral valve prolapse was the only cardiac condition found at necropsy (hereafter called isolated mitral valve prolapse); the remaining 41 patients had other conditions that were capable of being fatal. Of the latter 41 patients, 7, aged 17 to 59 years (mean 45), had associated congenital heart disease, and 34 patients, aged 17 to 70 years (mean 52), had no associated congenital cardiac abnormalities.

Compared with the 34 patients without associated congenital heart disease and with nonmitral valve prolapse conditions capable in themselves of being fatal, the 15 patients who died suddenly with isolated mitral valve prolapse were younger (mean age 39 ± 17 versus 52 ± 15 years; p = 0.01), more often women (67% versus 26%; p = 0.008) and had a lower frequency of mitral regurgitation (7% versus 38%; p = 0.02). The 15 patients dying suddenly with isolated mitral valve prolapse also were less likely to have evidence of ruptured chordae tendineae (29% versus 67%; p = 0.04).

The frequency of increased heart weight (67% versus 59%), a dilated mitral valve anulus (80% versus 81%), a dilated tricuspid valve anulus (17% versus 17%), an elongated anterior mitral leaflet (86% versus 54%), an elongated posterior mitral leaflet (79% versus 77%) and fibrous endocardial plaque under the posterior mitral leaflet (73% versus 63%) was similar between the two groups. The severity of the prolapse (mild 20% versus 11%; moderate 27% versus 58%; severe 53% versus 32%) also was similar between the two groups.

Thus, persons with mitral valve prolapse dying suddenly without another recognized condition tend to be relatively young women without mitral regurgitation.

(J Am Coll Cardiol 1991;17:921–31)

Mitral valve prolapse is a common condition affecting an estimated 5% of the U.S. population (1). A rare but much-feared occurrence in persons with mitral valve prolapse is sudden death. Although only a small number of patients with mitral valve prolapse die suddenly (without other potentially fatal conditions), mitral valve prolapse accounts for a substantial proportion of sudden deaths in persons without other clear causes of death. One study (2) of 50 persons, aged 7 to 35 years, dying suddenly and unexpectedly found mitral valve prolapse to be present in 12 (24%). Several necropsy studies (3–23) have reported on individuals or small groups of patients with sudden death associated with mitral valve prolapse.

No study has compared morphologic findings in patients with mitral valve prolapse unassociated with another potentially fatal condition (hereafter called isolated mitral valve prolapse) with those patients with mitral valve prolapse associated with another potentially fatal condition. Such a comparison is the purpose of this study.

Methods

Inclusion criteria. For a patient to be included in this study, three criteria had to be met: 1) the patient's heart was examined by the Pathology Branch, National Heart, Lung, and Blood Institute, and was classified by us as "mitral valve prolapse"; 2) at death, the patient was 16 to 70 years of age; and 3) the patient's heart (or photographs if the heart was unavailable) possessed morphologic features for the diagnosis of mitral valve prolapse used in this study (to be discussed subsequently). In cases where mitral valve replacement had been performed, the operatively excised mitral valve or photographs of it had to be available to reconfirm the diagnosis of mitral valve prolapse.

Sources of cases. From January 1956 to February 1990, the hearts of 101 patients were classified as "mitral valve prolapse" by the Pathology Branch, National Heart, Lung, and Blood Institute. Of these 101 heart specimens, 81 were available for reexamination by both authors and photographs of the hearts were available in the other 20 cases. Of the 101 cases, review of medical necropsy records disclosed that 21 patients were >70 years of age and that 2 were <16 years of

From the Pathology Branch, National Heart, Lung, and Blood Institute, National Institutes of Health, Bethesda, Maryland.

*Present address. Division of Cardiology, Department of Medicine, The Washington Hospital Center, Washington, DC.

Manuscript received August 7, 1990; revised manuscript received October 2, 1990, accepted October 14, 1990.

Address for reprints: William C. Roberts, MD. Pathology Branch, Building 10, Room 2N258, National Institutes of Health, Bethesda, Maryland 20892.

Table 1. Clinical and Morphologic Features of Mitral Valve Prolapse at Necropsy Unassociated With Other Congenital Cardiovascular Anomalies (49 patients aged 16 to 70 years)

Patient Category	+SCD −MR −CAD	+SCD +MR −CAD	+SCD −MR +CAD	−SCD +MR −CAD	−SCD −MR −CAD	Total (%)
No. of patients	14	3	3	10	19	49
Mean age (yr)	38 ± 17	50 ± 17	65 ± 3	55 ± 13	49 ± 17	48 ± 17
Women/men	10/4	0/3	0/3	3/7	6/13	19/30
Heart weight (g)	379 ± 96	770 ± 105	462 ± 103	577 ± 180	397 ± 131	458 ± 167
MV anulus >10 cm	11/14	1/1	2/3	8/8	6/10	29/36 (81)
TV anulus >14 cm	1/13	1/2	0/3	2/9	1/10	5/37 (14)
AML length >2.0 cm	11/13	1/1	2/3	2/4	3/6	19/27 (70)
PML length >1.5 cm	10/13	1/1	3/3	4/4	3/6	21/27 (78)
Absent chordae	4/12	0/1	2/2	6/8	2/6	14/29 (48)
LV cavity dilated (grade 3/4 or 4/4)	0/14	1/3	0/3	3/9	1/19	5/48 (10)
CA narrowed >75% in CSA	0/14	0/3	3/3	3/9	1/15	7/44 (16)
LV necrosis	0/14	0/3	1/3	0/10	0/18	1/48 (2)
LV fibrosis	0/14	1/3	1/3	2/10	1/18	5/48 (10)
Grade of MVP						
Mild	3/14	0/1	0/3	0/5	2/11	5/34 (15)
Moderate	4/14	0/1	2/3	2/5	7/11	15/34 (44)
Severe	7/14	1/1	1/3	3/5	2/11	14/34 (41)
Endocardial fibrous plaque under PML	10/14	1/1	1/3	6/7	5/9	23/34 (68)
Mitral annular calcium						
Grade 1–2/4	3/14	0/2	1/3	1/7	2/17	7/43 (16)
Grade 3–4/4	1/14	0/2	0/3	2/7	2/17	5/43 (12)
Valvular competent PFO	3/11	1/3	1/3	1/5	1/8	7/31 (23)
Redundant FO membrane	3/11	0/3	1/3	2/5	0/7	6/30 (20)
SCD due to MVP	14/14	1/3	0/3	0/10	0/19	15/49 (31)
The Marfan syndrome	2/14	0/3	0/3	2/10	4/19	8/49 (16)
Mitral valve replacement	0/14	2/3	0/3	1/10	0/19	3/49 (6)

AML = anterior mitral leaflet; CA = coronary artery; CAD = fatal coronary artery disease; CSA = cross-sectional area; FO = fossa ovale; LV = left ventricular; MR = severe mitral regurgitation; MV = mitral valve; MVP = mitral valve prolapse; PFO = patent foramen ovale; PML = posterior mitral leaflet; SCD = sudden cardiac death; TV = tricuspid valve; − = absent; + = present.

age and, therefore, these 23 cases were excluded. The children were excluded because morphologic comparisons with measurements in adults, such as heart weight, leaflet length and anular circumference, would be meaningless. Persons >70 years of age were excluded because some age-related changes in the mitral leaflets of elderly persons are similar to features of mitral valve prolapse, including leaflet thickening, especially in the portions adjacent to the posteromedial commissure, and the thickened portions often protrude toward the left atrium. Although several hearts in the elderly patients clearly had unequivocal features of mitral valve prolapse, many did not. To avoid including patients who did not have mitral valve prolapse, the older patients were excluded.

On reexamination of the remaining 78 patients, 22 were determined not to have morphologic features (to be discussed subsequently) of mitral valve prolapse. After these exclusions, 56 patients, aged 16 to 70 years (mean 48), remained and all had unequivocal morphologic features of mitral valve prolapse.

Definitions. *Sudden cardiac death* was defined as death occurring within 6 h of the onset of symptoms of cardiac dysfunction or myocardial ischemia. *Sudden death* associated with mitral valve prolapse (isolated mitral valve prolapse) was defined as sudden cardiac death where mitral valve prolapse was present and no other cardiac or noncardiac condition was present at autopsy to explain death. Sudden death associated with *coronary artery disease* was defined as sudden cardiac death with >75% cross-sectional area luminal narrowing of one or more of the four major epicardial coronary arteries. If both mitral valve prolapse and significant coronary arterial narrowing was present, death was attributed to coronary artery disease.

Significant mitral regurgitation was defined as the presence of at least "moderate" or grade 3/4 or 4/4 mitral regurgitation by left ventricular angiography or Doppler echocardiography. If no objective assessment of mitral regurgitation was made during life, significant mitral regurgitation was presumed to have been present if the left atrium and ventricle were significantly (grade >2/4) dilated in the absence of another cause of chamber enlargement.

Morphologic criteria of mitral valve prolapse. Morphologic criteria used for the diagnosis of mitral valve prolapse were: 1) elongation of a portion of the posterior mitral leaflet such that the distance from distal margin to its attachment at

Table 2. Clinical and Morphologic Features in 15 Patients Dying Suddenly Secondary to Mitral Valve Prolapse

Pt No.	Age (yr)	Race	Gender	MVP Diagnosed Clinically	The Marfan Syndrome	Location of Death	Last Activity	SC	SM	SH	CHF	VPCs on ECG	HW (g)	MV Anulus (cm)	TV Anulus (cm)	AML Length (cm)	PML Length (cm)	Chords Missing	Grade of MVP (1-3+)	Plaque Under PML	MAC (0-4+)	VC PFO	Redundant FO Membrane
1	16	W	M	+	+	Basketball court	Sitting after playing	-	+	0	0	+	325	12.5	12	3	2.5	+	2	0	0	-	-
2	18	W	F	+	0	Home	Arguing	-	0	0	0	+*	220	9.6	11.5	2	1.5	0	1	+	0	0	0
3	21	W	F	+	0	Work	Talking on phone	-	-	0	0	-	360	14	-	3	1.5	+	2	0	1	-	-
4	23	W	F	+	0	Work	Drinking water	+	+	0	0	-	280	10	9	2.5	2	0	3	+	0	+	+
5	26	W	F	+	0	Work	Talking	+	+	0	0	0†	265	12	11	3	3	0	3	+	0	+	+
6	40	B	M	0	0	Work	Sitting alone	-	-	-	0	-	570	15.5	13	3	2.5	0	3	+	0	0	0
7	30	W	M	0	0	Golf course	Playing golf	-	-	0	0	-	475	10	11	3	2	0	1	+	0	0	0
8	40	W	F	0	-	Home	Playing with children	-	-	0	0	-	355	13	12	-	-	+	2	0	2	-	+
9	47	W	F	0	0	Home	Gardening	-	-	0	0	+	445	12.5	12.5	2.5	2	0	3	+	0	0	0
10	51	W	M	+	0	Restaurant	Sitting after last dancing	+	+	0	0	0	500	10.5	12	2	1.5	0	1	0	0	0	0
11	53	W	F	+	0	Church	Sitting	-	-	0	0	+	325	12.6	10.5	2.5	3	0	2	+	3	0	0
12	53	W	F	0	0	Restaurant	Getting up to dance	-	-	-	0	-	390	13.6	11	3.5	3	0	3	+	1	+	+
13	55	W	F	+	0	Home	Standing	+	+	0	0	+	390	13	13	3	2.5	+	3	-	0	0	0
14	55	W	M	+	0	Home	Sleeping	-	+	0	+	+	670	>12	14	3.5	2	0	3	+	0	+	0
15	69	W	F	0	0	Home	—	-	-	-	0	-	400	15.4	14.5	2.5	3	+	3	+	0	0	0

*This patient had survived a cardiac arrest 2 years earlier; †this patient had a history of paroxysmal atrial tachycardia. AML = anterior mitral leaflet; B = black; CHF = congestive heart failure; F = female; FO = fossa ovale; HW = heart weight; M = male; MVP = mitral valve prolapse; MAC = mitral annular calcification; PFO = patent foramen ovale; PML = posterior mitral leaflet; Pt = patient; SC = systolic click; SH = systemic hypertension; SM = systolic murmur; TV = tricuspid valve; VC = valvular competent; VPC = ventricular premature complex; W = white; + = present; 0 = absent; - = no information available.

the mitral anulus was >1.5 cm; or 2) presence of mitral leaflet protrusion toward the left atrium, usually also associated with missing chordae tendineae, and the prolapsed portion of the leaflet involving >50% of the anterior leaflet and >33% of the posterior leaflet. Others (9,23) have referred to this leaflet prolapse as "interchordal hooding."

Morphologic measurements. All morphologic measurements and observations were performed by one or both authors. The length of the mitral leaflets was measured from the line of attachment of the leaflet to its free margin at the longest portion of each leaflet. Chordae tendineae were considered "missing" if none extended caudally from the ventricular surface of a portion of either or both leaflets or if detached chordae that had rounded or blunted distal ends were present. ("Missing" chordae were considered to represent sites of previously ruptured chordae [24]). The severity of mitral valve prolapse was subjectively graded as mild, moderate or severe.

Determination of normal measurement values. Normal values for various morphologic measurements were determined

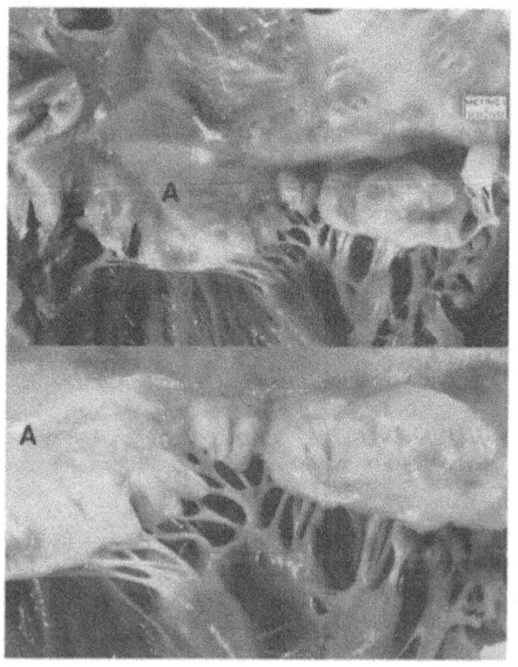

Figure 1. Patient 1. The heart of a 16 year old boy (Suffolk County Medical Examiner #84-4276, Hauppauge, NY) who had skeletal features of Marfan syndrome (examination of his aorta did not reveal "cystic medial necrosis"). He had a systolic murmur and mitral valve prolapse was diagnosed by echocardiography. His rest electrocardiogram showed occasional uniform premature ventricular complexes that disappeared with exercise. He died suddenly in a locker room after playing basketball. **Top,** View of the opened mitral valve, showing mild changes of mitral valve prolapse in the anterior leaflet (A) and more severe changes in the posterior leaflet. **Bottom,** Close-up view of the posterior leaflet.

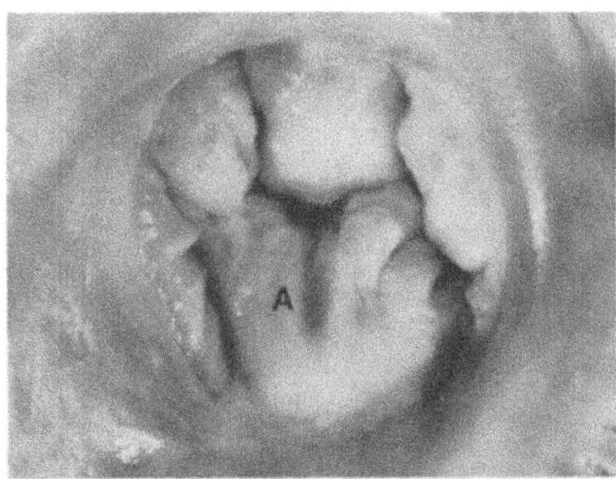

Figure 2. Patient 2. View of the intact mitral valve from the left atrium, showing a normal-appearing anterior leaflet (A) and prolapse of the posterior leaflets from the heart of an 18 year old woman (Rockford Memorial Hospital #A85-6, Rockford, IL) who was the daughter of a physician. Twenty-seven months before death, she had a cardiac arrest from which she was resuscitated. Evaluation included electrocardiography, coronary angiography, echocardiography, exercise stress testing, electrophysiologic studies and right ventricular endomyocardial biopsy. These examinations revealed mitral valve prolapse, a slightly prolonged QTc interval (0.46 s) and ventricular premature complexes that became more frequent and complex (couplets and triplets) during the recovery phase after exercise. She did not have mitral regurgitation. She was taking propranolol and mexiletine at the time of death, which occurred during an emotional argument.

by measurements in 20 normal hearts from persons aged 15 to 70 years (mean 47). The 95% confidence intervals derived from these measurements of normal hearts were: mitral anular circumference 7.8 to 8.5 cm, tricuspid valve anulus 8.4 to 11.4 cm, anterior mitral leaflet length 1.5 to 1.8 cm and posterior mitral leaflet length 1.1 to 1.3 cm. The following upper limits therefore were used: mitral anular circumference 10 cm; tricuspid valve anular circumference 14 cm; anterior mitral leaflet length 2 cm and posterior mitral length 1.5 cm.

Histologic studies. One or more of the following histologic sections (stained by hematoxylin and eosin or Movat stain) were prepared from each heart: 1) at least two sections of left ventricular myocardium extending from endocardium to epicardium; and 2) a transverse section of the ascending aorta about 1 cm cephalad to the sinotubular junction.

Results

Subgroupings of the patients with mitral valve prolapse without congenital heart disease. Table 1 summarizes clinical and morphologic findings in the 49 patients without congenital heart disease. The 49 patients were divided into five subgroups on the basis of the presence or absence of sudden cardiac death (SCD) (from any cause), regurgitation (MR) (as determined by objective studies during the patient's life

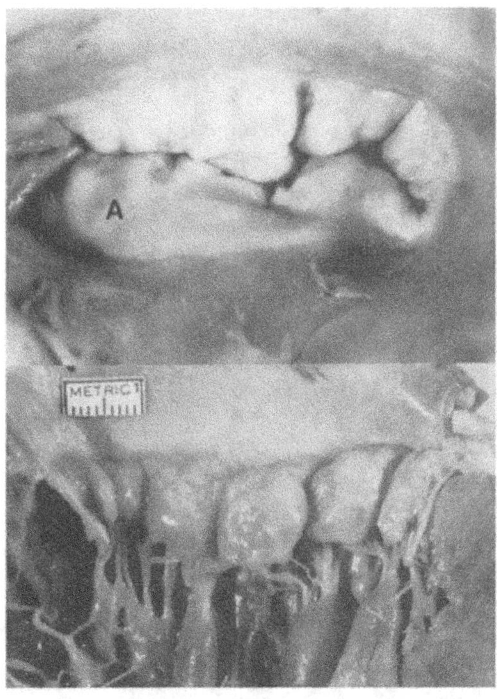

Figure 3. Patient 4. The heart of a 21 year old woman (York Hospital #81AX-132, York, PA) who had the diagnosis of mitral valve prolapse at age 16 years. One year before death, while pregnant, she complained of palpitation and substernal pressure. She died suddenly at a water fountain. **Top.** View of the intact mitral valve from the left atrium, showing prolapse of several scallops of the posterior leaflet, but the valve does not appear regurgitant. **Bottom.** View of the posterior leaflet of the opened mitral valve, showing extensive "hooding" and elongation of the leaflet. A = anterior leaflet.

and morphologic evidence of significant mitral regurgitation) and fatal coronary artery disease (CAD). Fourteen of the 15 patients who had sudden death associated with mitral valve prolapse (isolated mitral valve prolapse) comprise the category +SCD, −MR, −CAD, and the 1 patient with sudden death due to mitral valve prolapse but who had mitral regurgitation is in the category +SCD, −MR, −CAD. No patient had a history or morphologic evidence of infective endocarditis.

Characteristics of the 15 patients dying suddenly from mitral valve prolapse. Of the total group of 56 patients, 22 died suddenly from a cardiac cause: 4 had significant coronary artery disease (>75% cross-sectional area narrowing of at least one major epicardial coronary artery), 2 had had mitral valve replacement, 1 had cyanotic congenital heart disease and 15 (Table 2) had no explanation for death other than mitral valve prolapse. The age of the latter 15 patients ranged from 16 to 69 years (mean 39); 10 (67%) were women.

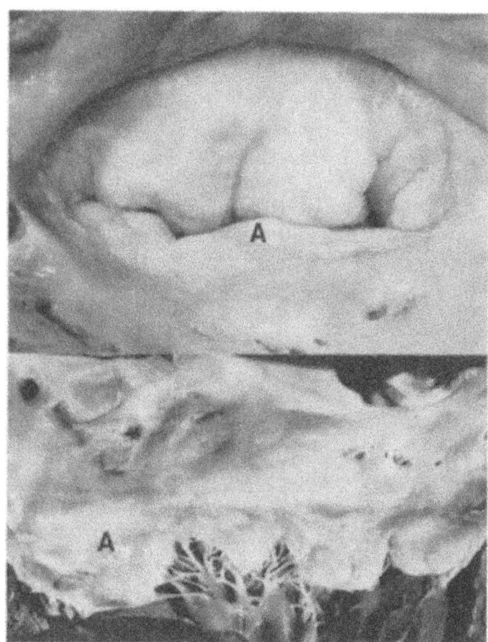

Figure 4. Patient 5. The heart of a 26 year old woman (District of Columbia Medical Examiner's Office #87-07-681) who was a lawyer. She had palpitation associated with paroxysmal atrial tachycardia beginning at age 9 years and had mitral valve prolapse diagnosed by echocardiography at age 15 years. She was started on propranolol therapy at 15 years of age and changed to atenolol 2 years before death. She had an episode of atrial tachycardia about once each 3 months, and it resolved promptly with the Valsalva maneuver. While talking with two colleagues she collapsed suddenly and died. **Top.** View of the intact mitral valve from the left atrium, showing pronounced prolapse of the posterior leaflet. **Bottom.** View of the opened mitral valve, showing pronounced "hooding" of the posterior leaflet. The anterior leaflet (A) is relatively uninvolved.

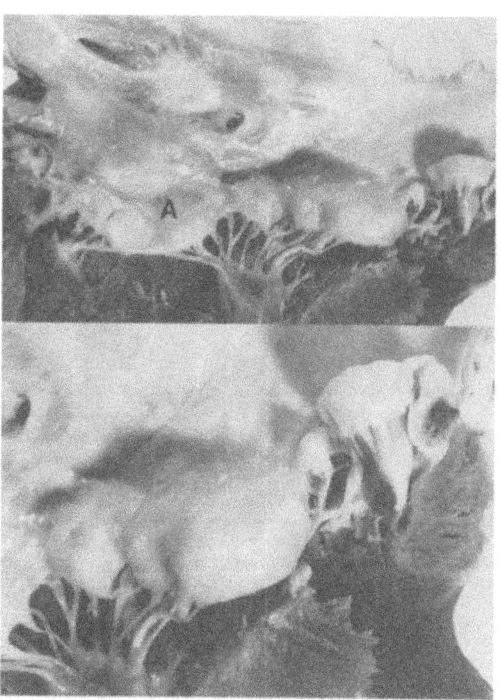

Figure 5. Patient 8. The heart of a 40 year old woman (Suffolk County Medical Examiner #84-4578, Hauppauge, NY) who had Marfan syndrome. She had a history of "valve problems," but no echocardiography was ever done. She was asymptomatic and on no medication. She collapsed suddenly and died while playing with neighborhood children. **Top.** View of the opened mitral valve, showing a mildly abnormal anterior leaflet (A) and a very abnormal posterior leaflet. **Bottom.** Close-up view of a portion of the posterior leaflet, showing a scallop of this leaflet, which is severely prolapsed toward the left atrium. This heart weighed 355 g and no chamber was dilated.

Diagnosis of mitral valve prolapse was made during life in eight (53%); Marfan syndrome was diagnosed in two (13%). Of seven patients whose electrocardiographic (ECG) data were available, six had ventricular premature complexes on their rest ECG, including one patient who had nonfatal cardiac arrest 2 years before death. Four patients were known to be on medication at the time of death: one woman who had nonfatal cardiac arrest was taking propranolol and mexiletine; one woman with paroxysmal atrial tachycardia was taking atenolol; one woman with frequent ventricular premature complexes was taking nadolol and one woman was taking thyroxine. Four patients died suddenly during or shortly after physical exertion and one patient died after an emotional argument.

Certain cardiac morphologic findings in some of the 15 patients who died suddenly from mitral valve prolapse are illustrated in Figures 1 to 7. In the 15 patients, the heart weight ranged from 220 to 670 g (mean 398); in the 5 men, four hearts weighed >400 g; in the 10 women, six hearts weighed >350 g. The mitral valve anulus was dilated (>10 cm in circumference) in 12 of the 15 patients (mean anular circumference 12.4 ± 1.9 cm). The anterior mitral leaflet was elongated (>2 cm from margin of attachment to free margin) in 12 of 14 patients, and the posterior leaflet was elongated (>1.5 cm) in 11 of 14 patients. In none of the 15 hearts was any major epicardial coronary artery narrowed >25% in cross-sectional area and none had gross or microscopic foci of myocardial necrosis or fibrosis. By visual inspection, the cardiac chambers were of normal size in eight patients, only mildly dilated in six and moderately dilated in one. Fibrous thickening of the mural endocardium (endocardial plaque) behind the posterior mitral leaflet was present in 11 of the 15 patients. The presence or absence of mitral

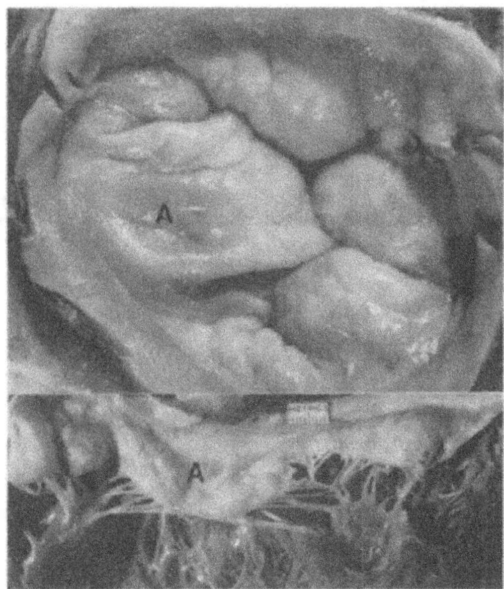

Figure 6. Patient 9. The heart of a 47 year old woman (District of Columbia Medical Examiner's Office #80-06-485) who was a psychiatrist. She had been dieting for 2 weeks before death and was taking thyroid supplements to aid in her weight loss. She was found dead in her yard, dressed in jogging clothes. Her only known cardiac problem was ventricular premature complexes noted by her physician husband. **Top.** View of the intact mitral valve from the left atrium, showing both the anterior (A) and posterior leaflets to be redundant. **Bottom.** The opened mitral valve, showing the posterior leaflet to be elongated.

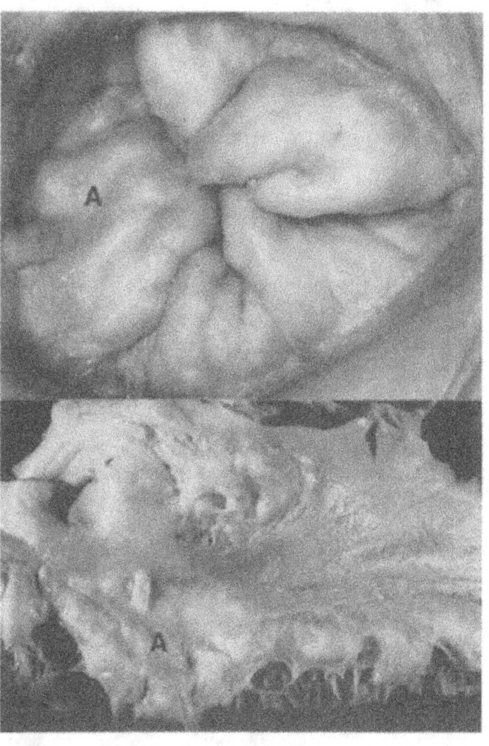

Figure 7. Patient 12. The heart of a 53 year old woman (District of Columbia Medical Examiner's Office #88-09-961) who was the wife of a plastic surgeon. She was out with her husband, got up to dance and suddenly collapsed and died. **Top.** View of the intact mitral valve from the left atrium, showing prolapse of the posterior leaflet above the anterior leaflet (A). **Bottom.** The opened mitral valve, showing a very large anterior leaflet (A) and an elongated redundant posterior leaflet.

regurgitation was documented during life by objective testing in three patients: echocardiography showed trace mitral regurgitation in one patient; left ventricular angiography showed no regurgitation in one patient and moderate regurgitation in another. The latter patient's heart weighed 670 g and all four cardiac chambers were moderately dilated.

Comparison of patients dying suddenly with isolated mitral valve prolapse with other patients with mitral valve prolapse without congenital heart disease. Comparison of the 15 patients in whom sudden death was associated with isolated mitral valve prolapse (14 patients from the group $-SCD$, $-MR$, $-CAD$ and 1 patient with mitral regurgitation from the group $+SCD$, $+MR$, $-CAD$) with the other patients with mitral valve prolapse without associated congenital heart disease (Table 1) disclosed the following differences: 1) a lower mean age at death (39 ± 17 versus 52 ± 15 years; p = 0.01); 2) a preponderance of women (10 [67%] of 15 versus 9 [26%] of 34; p = 0.008); 3) a lower frequency of mitral regurgitation (1 [7%] of 15 versus 13 [38%] of 34; p = 0.02); and 4) a lower frequency of having evidence of ruptured chordae tendineae (4 [29%] of 14 versus 10 [67%] of 15; p = 0.04). No significant differences were noted between the

patients dying suddenly with mitral valve prolapse and the other patients with mitral valve prolapse with regard to heart weight, circumference of the mitral or tricuspid anulus, length of the anterior or posterior mitral leaflet, presence of missing chordae tendineae, grade of mitral valve prolapse, presence of endocardial fibrous plaque under the posterior mitral leaflet or presence of a patent foramen ovale or redundant fossa ovale membrane. Cardiac morphologic findings in two patients from the group $-SCD$, $+MR$, $-CAD$ are illustrated in Figures 8 and 9 and two patients from the group $-SCD$, $-MR$, $-CAD$ are illustrated in Figures 10 and 11.

Mitral valve prolapse associated with congenital heart disease. Congenital heart disease was present in 7 of the 56 patients (Table 3). These congenital abnormalities included *ostium secundum atrial septal defect* (four patients), *bicuspid aortic valve* (three patients), *coarctation of the aorta* (one patient), *Ebstein's anomaly* (one patient), *partial atrio-*

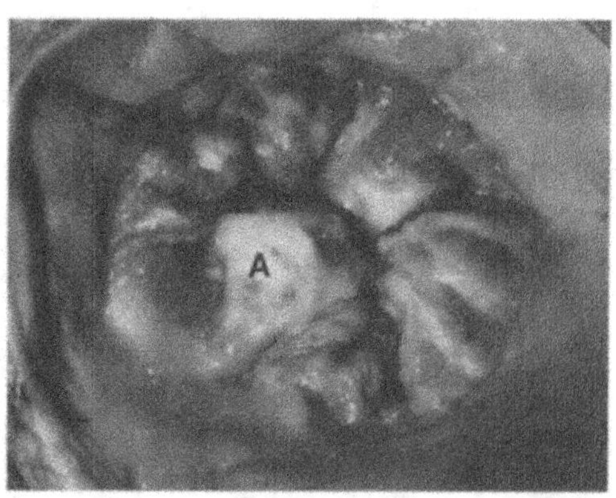

Figure 8. Patient from $-SCD$, $+MR$, $-CAD$ group. The heart of a 65 year old woman (Georgetown University Hospital #81A-122, Washington, DC) who had chronic congestive heart failure and severe mitral regurgitation. She died in cardiogenic shock. View of the intact mitral valve from the left atrium, showing prolapse of both the anterior (A) and posterior mitral leaflets. CAD = fatal coronary artery disease; MR = mitral regurgitation; SCD = sudden cardiac death; − = absent; + = present.

ventricular canal (one patient) and *sinus of Valsalva aneurysm* (one patient). The patient with total anomalous pulmonary venous connection and one patient with a severely stenotic bicuspid aortic valve died suddenly.

Mitral valve prolapse associated with the Marfan syndrome. Eight patients had the Marfan syndrome, two of whom died suddenly without a clear cause. Three had rupture of the ascending aorta, one had congestive heart failure with severe aortic and mitral regurgitation and two died of noncardiac causes. Histologic sections of ascending aorta were available in six of the eight patients: four had

Figure 9. Patient from $-SCD$, $+MR$, $-CAD$ group. The heart of a 54 year old man (District of Columbia Veterans Administration Hospital #83A-84, Washington, DC) with grade 3/4 chronic atrial fibrillation and mitral regurgitation by ventriculography. He died of a cerebral embolic event. **a.** View of the intact mitral valve from the left atrium, showing a patulous mitral valve with a very dilated anulus (15 cm). **b.** Close-up view of the posterior leaflet of the opened mitral valve, showing pronounced hooding of each of the scallops of the leaflet. **c.** The opened mitral valve. **d.** Transverse slices of the ventricles, showing a surprising lack of left ventricular dilation given the degree of mitral regurgitation present. Abbreviations as in Figure 8.

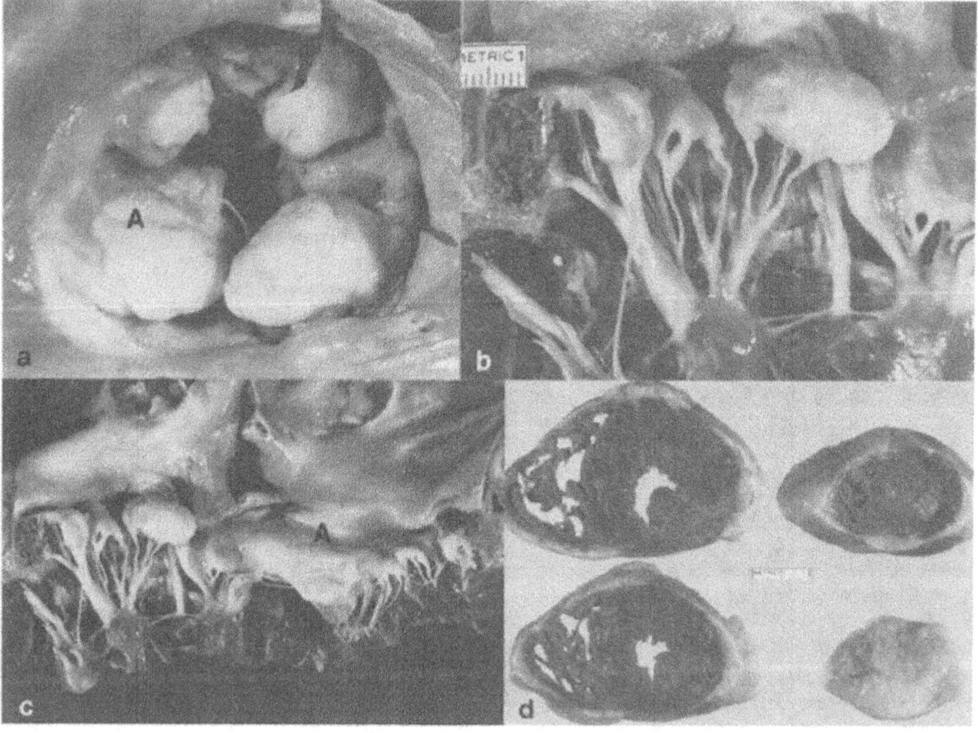

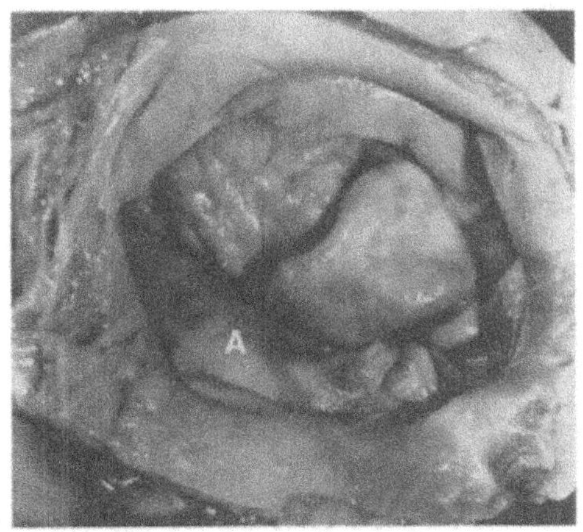

Figure 10. Patient from −*SCD*, −*MR*, −*CAD* group. The heart of a 63 year old woman (Georgetown University Hospital #79A-100, Washington, D.C.) who died of cancer. View of the intact mitral valve from the left atrium, showing herniation of the posterior leaflet above the anterior leaflet (A). Abbreviations as in Figure 8.

classic "medial cystic necrosis" with massive degeneration of elastic fibers and two had a normal configuration of elastic fibers in the aortic media. At least one histologic section of ascending aorta stained for elastic fibers was examined in 22 patients with mitral valve prolapse unassociated with the Marfan syndrome, and the aortic media in each appeared normal.

Discussion

Major findings in the present study. Several differences were observed in the 15 patients with sudden death associated with isolated mitral valve prolapse (without the pres-

Figure 11. Patient from −*SCD*, −*MR*, −*CAD* group. The heart of a 63 year old man (Georgetown University Hospital #82A-04, Washington, DC) who died of cancer. a. View of the heart from above after removal of the atria. b. Radiograph of the base of the heart, showing massive calcium deposits in the anulus of the mitral valve, aortic valve and epicardial coronary arteries. c. Close-up view of the intact mitral valve as viewed from the left atrium showing pronounced enlargement of the posterior leaflet. d. View of the aortic valve from above, showing a stenotic tricuspid valve with calcium deposits and no fusion of the commissures. Abbreviations as in Figure 8.

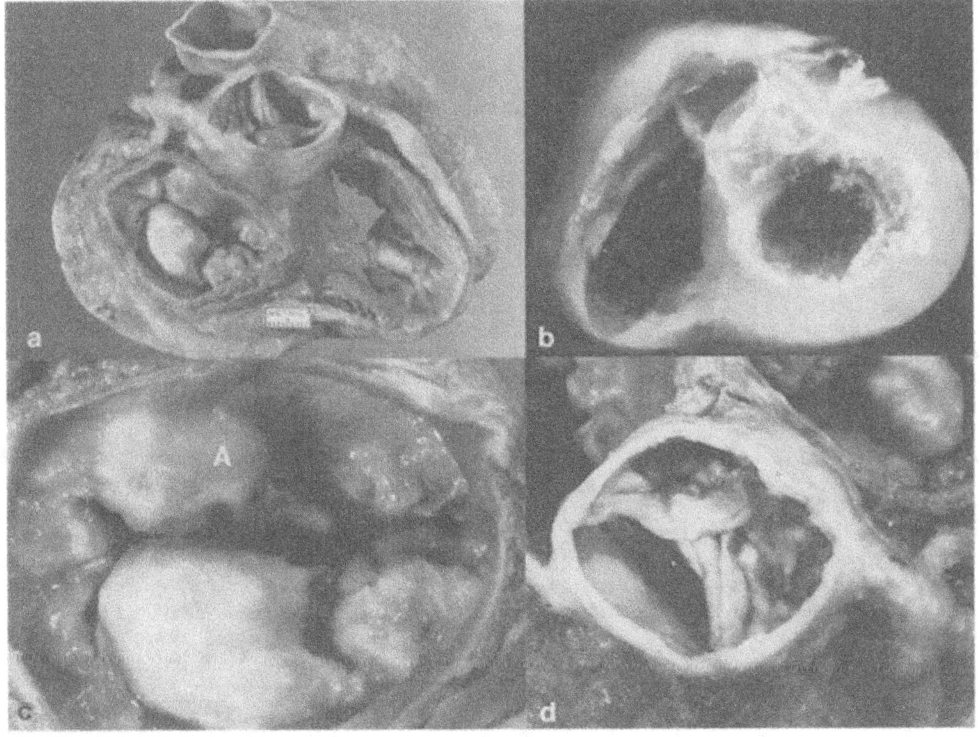

Table 3. Clinical Features of Seven Adult Patients With Congenital Heart Disease With Morphologic Features of Mitral Valve Prolapse Studied at Necropsy

Pt No.	Congenital Abnormality	Age (yr), Gender	MVP Diagnosed Clinically	MR	Cardiac Operation	Mode of Death
1	ASD (secundum), Ebstein's anomaly	17 F	0	·	0	Noncardiac (cancer)
2	Aortic coarctation, BAV (AR)	30 M	+	·	Coarctectomy, AVR, MVR	Cardiac operation
3	ASD (secundum), TAPVC	42 M	0	·	0	Sudden (cardiac)
4	Atrioventricular canal (partial)	55 F	+	·	0	Noncardiac (pneumonia)
5	BAV, valvular aortic stenosis	56 M	—		Coronary bypass	Sudden (CAD + AS)
6	ASD (secundum), BAV, SV aneurysm	57 F	0	·	0	Rupture of SV aneurysm
7	ASD (secundum)	59 F	+	+	ASD closure, MVR	Cardiac operation

ASD = atrial septal defect, AVR = aortic valve replacement, BAV = bicuspid aortic valve, MVR = mitral valve replacement; SV = sinus of Valsalva; TAPVC = total anomalous pulmonary venous connection. + = present; 0 = absent. · = no information available; other abbreviations as in Tables 1 and 2.

ence of other potentially fatal conditions) compared with the patients with mitral valve prolapse with other potentially fatal causes of death and without other congenital cardiac malformations: the patients who died suddenly with isolated mitral valve prolapse were younger, more likely to be women and less likely to have mitral regurgitation or evidence of ruptured chordae tendineae.

Severe mitral regurgitation was infrequent (1 of 15 patients) in the patients with mitral valve prolapse who died suddenly without associated significant coronary artery disease or other congenital cardiac anomalies. There have been conflicting views regarding the importance of mitral regurgitation as a predisposing factor for sudden death in patients with mitral valve prolapse. Some investigators (25,26) emphasized the importance of mitral regurgitation as a risk factor for sudden death in patients with mitral valve prolapse, going so far as to calculate an estimated annual mortality rate from sudden death due to mitral valve prolapse in patients with and without mitral regurgitation. Their estimates were based primarily on a study by Davies et al. (15), who reported on 13 patients at necropsy who died suddenly and had mitral valve prolapse. At least 4 of their 13 patients, however, had an etiology for the mitral regurgitation and sudden death other than mitral valve prolapse: 2 patients had bacterial endocarditis, 1 had a previous myocardial infarction and 1 patient, a 79 year old man, had chronic lung disease. After reviewing 25 previously reported patients with mitral valve prolapse who died suddenly, Jeresaty (27) concluded that the typical patient with mitral valve prolapse who dies suddenly has only minimal to moderate mitral regurgitation.

Frequency of mural endocardial fibrous plaque in patients dying suddenly with mitral valve prolapse. The presence of mural endocardial fibrous plaque beneath the posterior mitral leaflet has been noted previously in necropsy studies of patients dying suddenly from mitral valve prolapse. Chesler et al. (22) suggested that the friction between chordae tendineae and the underlying left ventricular mural endocardium, presumably the mechanism of formation of this endocardial plaque, may cause ventricular arrhythmias. We found a high frequency of such plaque, both in patients

whose death was attributed to isolated mitral valve prolapse (11 of 15) and patients whose death was attributed to other causes (12 of 19).

Abnormalities of the fossa ovale membrane in patients with mitral valve prolapse. Secundum atrial septal defect is associated with mitral valve prolapse (28,29). Four of our seven patients with mitral valve prolapse and congenital heart disease had ostium secundum atrial septal defect. Redundancy (aneurysm) of the fossa ovale membrane also has been noted (30) in association with mitral valve prolapse at necropsy, and a recent report (31) found a higher prevalence of atrial septal aneurysm diagnosed by echocardiography in patients with mitral valve prolapse (9.5%) compared with those without (3.1%). We found a 20% frequency of redundancy of the fossa ovale membrane among the 49 patients with mitral valve prolapse without congenital cardiovascular anomalies. Probe-patent valvular-competent foramen ovale occurred in 7 (23%) of 31 patients among the entire group. This frequency, however, is similar to that of valvular-competent patent foramen ovale in normal adult hearts (30). Neither redundancy of the fossa ovale membrane nor probe-patency of the foramen ovale was more common among the sudden death group compared with the other patients with mitral valve prolapse.

Previously reported studies on patients who died suddenly from mitral valve prolapse. We searched for published reports of patients with mitral valve prolapse who died suddenly and who had no other condition present at autopsy to explain death. A total of 63 patients (3–14,16–23) were found, of whom 39 had individualized clinical data (3–14, 16–22) (Table 4). These previously reported patients were similar in many respects to our group of 15 patients dying suddenly with mitral valve prolapse. The mean age of the previously published patients was 33 ± 14 years; 27 (71%) of 38 were women and the mean heart weight was 306 ± 76 g. Severe mitral regurgitation was uncommon; only one patient had a heart weight above normal (≤350 g for women and ≤400 g for men) and only one other patient (whose heart weighed 340 g) had dilated cardiac chambers. Only six patients had results of cineangiocardiography: mitral regur-

Table 4. Clinical Information in 39 Previously Reported Patients Studied at Necropsy Who Died Suddenly With Mitral Valve Prolapse as the Only Explanation for Death

Reference (first author)	Year	Age (yr)/ Gender	MVP Diagnosed Clinically	P	D	S	CP	MR	SH	CHF	SC	SM	MR by LV Cine (0–3+)	Rhythm	QTc (ms)	T Wave Inversion	VPCs	Last Activity	Medication	HW (g)	AML	PML	Plaque Under PML
Hancock (3)	1966	29/F	+	+	0	0	0	–	0	0	+	+	–	S	45	+(A,I)	+	—	Quinidine	–	–	–	–
Barlow (4)	1968	39/M	+	–	–	–	–		–	–	+	+	–	–	–	–	+	Mowing lawn	—	–	–	–	–
Trent (5)	1970	63/F	+	+	0	0	+	Y	0	+	0	+	++	S	–	–	0	—	Digoxin	340	+	+	–
Jeresaty (6)	1973	62/F	+	–	–	–	–	–	–	–	0	+	++	AF	N	+(A,I)	+	Sleeping	—	–	–	–	–
Shappell (7)	1973	27/F	+	0	0	+	0	N	0	0	+	+	0	S	45–47	+(I)	0	Arguing	Propranolol	310	+	+	–
Marshall (8)	1974	36/F	+	+	+	0	0	–	0	0	–	–	–	–	–	–	–	Sitting		350	+	+	–
Guthrie* (9)	1976	20/F	+	0	0	0	0		–	0	+	0	–		N	0	+	—	0	–	–	–	–
Guthrie* (9)	1976	25/F	+	+	+	+	+		–	–	+	+	+	–	–	–	+	—	Quinidine, propranolol	–	–	–	–
Guthrie* (9)	1976	29/M	0	0	0	0	0		–	0	0	+	–	–	–	–	–	Sitting at desk	—	–	–	–	–
Jeresaty (10)	1976	39/F	+	0	0	0	0	Y	0	0	+	+	+	S	N	+(I)	0	—	Furosemide	–	+	+	–
Kleid (11)	1976	38/F	–	+	0	0	0	N	0	0	0	+	–	S	–	–	+	—	0	–	–	–	–
Koch (12)	1976	9/–	+	–	–	–	–	–	–	–	–	–	–	–	–	–	••	—	—	–	–	–	–
Koch (12)	1976	30/–	+	–	–	–	–	–	–	–	–	–	–	–	–	–	••	—	—	–	–	–	–
Koch (12)	1976	32/–	+	–	–	–	–	–	–	–	–	–	–	–	–	–	••	—	—	–	–	–	–
Koch (12)	1976	50/–	+	–	–	–	–	–	–	–	–	–	–	–	–	–	••	—	—	–	–	–	–
Koch (12)	1976	64/–	+	–	–	–	–	–	–	–	–	–	–	–	–	–	••	—	—	–	–	–	–
Mills (14)	1977	58/M	+	–	+	–	–	–	–	+	0	+	–	–	–	+	+	—	Quinidine	–	–	–	–
Mair (16)	1980	25/F	+	+	0	+	0	–	0	0	+	+	–	–	–	–	–	Driving	0	230	+	+	+
Mair (16)	1980	29/F	+	–	–	+	–	–	0	0	+	0	–	–	–	–	–	Lying in bed	0	250	+	+	+
Mair (16)	1980	35/F	–	+	+	0	0	–	0	0	–	–	–	–	–	–	–	Conversing	0	270	+	+	+
Bharati (17)	1981	17/M	0	–	–	–	–	–	–	0	–	–	–	–	–	–	–	Playing football	—	–	–	–	–
Bharati (17)	1981	19/F	0	–	–	–	–	–	–	–	–	–	–	–	–	–	–	—	—	–	–	–	–
Bharati (18)	1981	45/M	+	+	–	–	–	–	–	–	+	+	–	S	N	–	+	—	0	–	–	+	–
Dupasquier (19)	1981	43/M	+	+		+	0	Y	0	0	0	+	–	S	N	+(I)	0	Driving	0	550	–	–	–
Salmela (20)	1981	27/M	+	–	+	+	0	–	0	0	+	+	–	S	N	+(I)	+	Watching television	Digoxin	–	–	+	–
Pocock (21)	1984	24/F	+	+	0	0	0	Y	0	0	+	+	+	S	N	+(I)	+	Conversing	Disopromide, acebutolol	–	0	+	+
Chesler (22)	1983	14/F	0	0	0	0	0	0	–	–	–	–	–	–	–	–	–	—	Methyldopa	230	+	+	+
Chesler (22)	1983	19/F	–	–	–	–	–	–	–	–	–	–	–	–	–	–	–	—	—	230	0	–	+
Chesler (22)	1983	19/M	+	0	0	0	0	0	–	–	+	+	–	–	–	–	–	—	Steroid inhaler	220	+	–	+
Chesler (22)	1983	21/F	+	0	0	0	0	0	–	–	+	0	–	–	–	–	–	—	Primidone	260	0	–	0
Chesler (22)	1983	21/F	+	+	0	0	0	0	–	–	+	+	–	–	–	–	–	—	0	290	+	–	+
Chesler (22)	1983	24/F	–	0	0	0	0	0	–	–	0	+	–	–	–	–	–	—	0	350	+	–	+
Chesler (22)	1983	25/F	+	+	+	0	+		–	–	+	+	–	–	–	–	–	—	Propranolol	220	+	–	+
Chesler (22)	1983	26/F	–	–	–	–	–	–	–	–	–	–	–	–	–	–	–	—	—	340	+	+	+
Chesler (22)	1983	27/F	–	0	0	0	0	0	–	–	0	+	–	–	–	–	–	—	0	325	+	+	+
Chesler (22)	1983	29/M	–	+	0	0	0	0	–	–	0	+	–	–	–	–	–	—	0	365	–	+	+
Chesler (22)	1983	30/M	+	0	0	0	0	0	–	–	+	0	–	–	–	–	–	—	0	325	+	+	+
Chesler (22)	1983	39/F	0	0	0	0	0	0	–	–	0	0	–	–	–	–	–	—	0	348	+	+	0
Chesler (22)	1983	59/F	0	0	0	0	0	0	–	–	–	–	–	–	–	–	–	—	0	320	0	+	+

*Some of the details of these cases were not in the original report but were provided in Jeresaty (6); two of these five patients had multiform ventricular premature complexes (VPCs) on their electrocardiogram. A = anterior; AF = atrial fibrillation; CP = chest pain; D = dizziness; I = inferior; LV Cine = left ventricular cineangiogram; N = normal; P = palpitation; QTc = QT interval corrected for rate; S = syncope; Y = yes; other abbreviations as in Tables 1 and 2.

gitation was absent in one, mild in three and moderate in two.

Previously reported patients with mitral valve prolapse who survived potentially lethal ventricular arrhythmias. Several studies (33–35) have detailed the characteristics of patients with mitral valve prolapse who had life-threatening ventricular tachyarrhythmias or who survived cardiac arrest. Winkle et al. (33) reported on seven patients (five women, mean age 49 years) with mitral valve prolapse who had survived one or more episodes of life-threatening ventricular arrhythmias: six patients had a systolic click or systolic murmur, or both. Mitral regurgitation was objectively diagnosed or excluded in only three of the seven patients (by left ventricular angiography): mitral regurgitation was absent in two and moderate in one. Wei et al. (34) reported on 10 patients with mitral valve prolapse (7 women, mean age 47 years) with symptomatic recurrent ventricular tachyarrhythmias refractory to conventional drug therapy. Although left ventricular angiography was performed in all patients, there was no specific mention of mitral regurgitation. Boudoulas et al. (35) reported on nine patients with mitral valve prolapse who had cardiac arrest (seven women, mean age 33 years) of whom seven survived. All seven had cardiac catheterization, but mitral regurgitation was not mentioned.

References

1. Savage DD, Garrison RJ, Devereux RB, et al. Mitral valve prolapse in the general population. I. Epidemiologic features: the Framingham Study. Am Heart J 1983;106:571–6.
2. Topaz O, Edwards JE. Pathologic features of sudden death in children, adolescents, and young adults. Chest 1985;87:476–82.
3. Hancock EW, Cohn K. The syndrome associated with midsystolic click and late systolic murmur. Am J Med 1966;41:183–96.
4. Barlow JB, Bosman CK, Pocock WA, Marchand P. Late systolic murmurs and non-ejection ("mid-late") systolic clicks: an analysis of 90 patients. Br Heart J 1968;30:203–18.
5. Trent JK, Adelman AG, Wigle ED, Silverman MD. Morphology of a prolapsed posterior mitral valve leaflet. Am Heart J 1970;79:539–43.
6. Jeresaty RM. Mitral valve prolapse-click syndrome. Prog Cardiovasc Dis 1973;15:623–52.
7. Shappell SD, Marshall CE, Brown RE, Bruce T. Sudden death and the familial occurrence of mid-systolic click, late systolic murmur syndrome. Circulation 1973;48:1128–34.
8. Marshall CE, Shappell SD. Sudden death and the ballooning posterior leaflet syndrome: detailed anatomic and histochemical investigation. Arch Pathol 1974;98:134–8.
9. Guthrie RB, Edwards JE. Pathology of the myxomatous mitral valve nature, secondary changes and complications. Minn Med 1976;59:637–47.
10. Jeresaty RM. Sudden death and the mitral valve prolapse-click syndrome. Am J Cardiol 1976;37:317–8.
11. Kleid JJ. Sudden death and the floppy mitral valve syndrome. Angiology 1976;27:734–7.
12. Koch FH, Hancock EW. Ten year follow-up of forty patients with the mid-systolic click/late systolic murmur syndrome (abstr). Am J Cardiol 1976;37:149.
13. Allen H, Harris A, Leatham A. Significance and prognosis of an isolated late systolic murmur: a 9-to-22-year follow-up. Br Heart J 1974;36:525–32.
14. Mills P, Rose J, Hollingsworth J, Amara I, Craige E. Long-term prognosis of mitral-valve prolapse. N Engl J Med 1977;297:13–8.
15. Davies MJ, Moore BP, Braimbridge MV. The floppy mitral valve: study of incidence, pathology, and complications in surgical, necropsy, and forensic material. Br Heart J 1978;40:468–81.
16. Mair WJ. Sudden death in young females with floppy mitral valve syndrome. Aust N Z J Med 1980;10:221–3.
17. Bharati S, Granston AS, Liebson PR, Loeb HS, Rosen KM, Lev M. The conduction system in mitral valve prolapse syndrome with sudden death. Am Heart J 1981;101:667–70.
18. Bharati S, Rosen KM, Miller LB, Strasberg B, Lev M. Sudden death in three teenagers (abstr). Circulation 1981;64(suppl IV):IV-72.
19. Dupasquier E, Berney JL. Le syndrome du prolapsus valvulaire mitral: deux complications rares: la mort subite, l'embolie cerebrale. Schweiz Med Wochenschr 1981;111:73–81.
20. Salmela PI, Ikaheimo M, Juustila H. Fatal ventricular fibrillation after treatment with digoxin in a 27-year-old man with mitral leaflet prolapse syndrome. Br Heart J 1981;46:338–41.
21. Pocock W, Bosman CK, Chesler E, Barlow JB, Edwards JE. Sudden death in primary mitral valve prolapse. Am Heart J 1984;107:378–82.
22. Chesler E, King RA, Edwards JE. The myxomatous mitral valve and sudden death. Circulation 1983;67:632–9.
23. Virmani R, Atkinson JB, Forman MB, Rabinowitz M. Mitral valve prolapse. Hum Pathol 1987;18:596–602.
24. Roberts WC, McIntosh CL, Wallace RB. Mechanisms of severe mitral regurgitation in mitral valve prolapse determined from analysis of operatively excised valves. Am Heart J 1987;113:1316–23.
25. Kligfield P, Levy D, Devereux RB, Savage DD. Arrhythmias and sudden death in mitral valve prolapse. Am Heart J 1987;113:1298–307.
26. Devereux RB, Kramer-Fox R, Kligfield P. Mitral valve prolapse: causes, clinical manifestations, and management. Ann Intern Med 1989;111:305–17.
27. Jeresaty RM. Mitral Valve Prolapse. New York: Raven, 1979:209–21.
28. Betriu A, Wigle ED, Felderhof CH, McLoughlin MJ. Prolapse of the posterior leaflet of the mitral valve associated with secundum atrial septal defect. Am J Cardiol 1975;35:363–9.
29. Leachman RD, Cokkinos DV, Cooley DA. Association of ostium secundum septal defects with mitral valve prolapse. Am J Cardiol 1976;38:167–9.
30. Roberts WC. Aneurysm (redundancy) of the atrial septum (fossa ovale membrane) and prolapse (redundancy) of the mitral valve. Am J Cardiol 1984;54:1153–4.
31. Rahko PS, Xu QB. Increased prevalence of atrial septal aneurysm in mitral valve prolapse (abstr). Circulation 1989;80(suppl II):II-10.
32. Barry A, Patten BM. The structure of the adult heart. In: Gould SE, ed. Pathology of the Heart and Blood Vessels. Springfield, IL: Charles C Thomas, 1968:91–130.
33. Winkle RA, Lopes MG, Popp RL, Hancock EW. Life-threatening arrhythmias in the mitral valve prolapse syndrome. Am J Med 1976;60:961–7.
34. Wei JY, Bulkley BH, Schaeffer AH, Greene HL, Reid PR. Mitral-valve prolapse syndrome and recurrent ventricular tachyarrhythmias. Ann Intern Med 1978;89:6–9.
35. Boudoulas H, Schaal SF, Stang JM, Fontana ME, Kolibash AJ, Wooley CF. Mitral valve prolapse-sudden death with long term survival (abstr). J Am Coll Cardiol 1986;7:29A.

Prolonged Survival (74 Years) in Unoperated Tetralogy of Fallot with Associated Mitral Valve Prolapse

Daniel J. Fernicola, MD, Victor R. Boodhoo, MD, and William C. Roberts, MD

Prolonged survival in tetralogy of Fallot is rare. About 5% of patients without operative therapy 5% survive >25 years. Recently, we studied at necropsy a man with tetralogy of Fallot who survived 74 years without operation and at necropsy severe mitral valve prolapse also was present. A description of pertinent findings in him are described herein.

S.D., a 74-year-old white man, who worked in a post office as a mail sorter, was cyanotic at birth and had recurrent syncope until the age of 8 years. He was then asymptomatic until age 43 when he developed numbness in his left hand and it recurred. At age 46, the first of 2 cardiac catheterizations was performed and the results are summarized in Table I. Atrial fibrillation began at age 58, and left ventriculogram at age 68 disclosed moderate mitral regurgitation. From age 46 to 55 he had episodic upper gastrointestinal tract bleeding from a gastric ulcer, and on 1 occasion his blood hematocrit was reduced to 24%. Signs and symptoms of congestive heart failure began at age 73, about 17 months before death. Examination at that time disclosed a grade 4/6 systolic murmur, loudest along the upper left sternal border. His fingers and toes were clubbed and cyanotic. The blood hematocrit was 36% and the systemic oxygen saturation was 80%. An electrocardiogram showed atrial fibrillation, incomplete right bundle branch block, right ventricular hypertrophy, and nonspecific ST-T-wave changes (Figure 1). He died of progressive congestive heart failure.

At necropsy, the heart weighed 860 g and the typical features of tetralogy of Fallot, namely ventricular septal defect and right ventricular outflow obstruction were present (Figures 2 and 3). Both mitral leaflets were thickened and both, the posterior more than the anterior, protruded abnormally into the left atrium. Only 1 coronary ostium was present in the aorta and it was located in the left aortic sinus (Figure 4). A radiograph of the heart specimen disclosed heavy calcific deposits in the left circumflex and in its continuation as the right coronary artery, but insignificant luminal narrowing was present (Figure 5). The epicardial coronary arteries were much more dilated than expected (for age 74 years). All 76 five-mm segments of the epicardial coronary arteries were narrowed <50% in cross-sectional area despite heavy calcific deposits within some portions of the walls.

This patient had classic tetralogy of Fallot with a large ventricular septal defect and severe subpulmonic and pulmonic valve obstruction. The pulmonic valve had a unicuspid structure. Additionally, the patient had a single coronary ostium in the aorta, and the very dilated epicardial coronary arteries were devoid of significant narrowing despite

From the Pathology Branch, National Heart, Lung, and Blood Institute, National Institutes of Health, Bethesda, Maryland, and the Parrish Medical Center, Titusville, Florida. Manuscript received August 18, 1992; revised manuscript received and accepted September 21, 1992.

TABLE I Cardiac Catheterization Data in the Patient Described

Site	Age (years) at Study 46	Age (years) at Study 68
Right atrium (mean) (mm Hg)	6	10
Right ventricle (s/d) (mm Hg)	95/0 } psg = 70	105/10 } psg = 70
Pulmonary artery (s/d) (mm Hg)	25/0	35/12
Pulmonary artery wedge (mean) (mm Hg)	16	21
Left ventricle (s/d) (mm Hg)	—	105/15
Systemic artery (s/d) (mm Hg)	110/50	105/70
Systemic O₂ saturation (%)	89	83
Blood hematocrit (%)	49	40*
Coronary angiogram	—	Single ostium

*Hospitalized for upper gastrointestinal bleed 5 months before catheterization.
O₂ = oxygen; psg = peak systolic gradient; s/d = peak systole/end diastole.

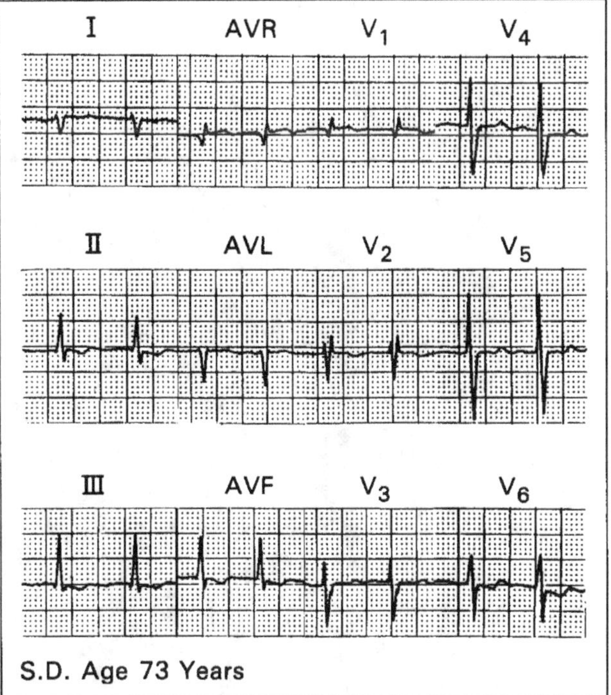

FIGURE 1. Electrocardiogram of the patient recorded 17 months before death.

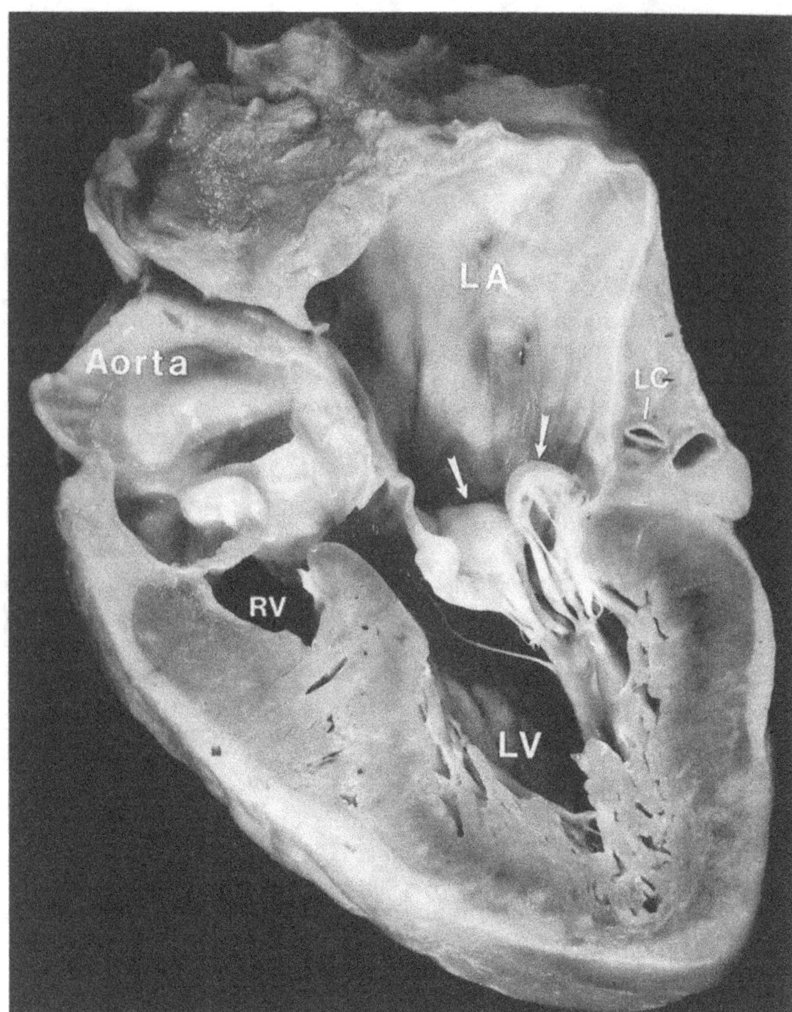

FIGURE 2. The heart at necropsy after an anteroposterior longitudinal cut. The ventricular septal defect is located just caudal to the overriding aorta. The right ventricular (RV) outflow tract is narrowed. Both mitral leaflets (arrows) prolapse into the dilated left atrium (LA). The left ventricular (LV) cavity is moderately dilated. The left circumflex (LC) coronary artery is very dilated.

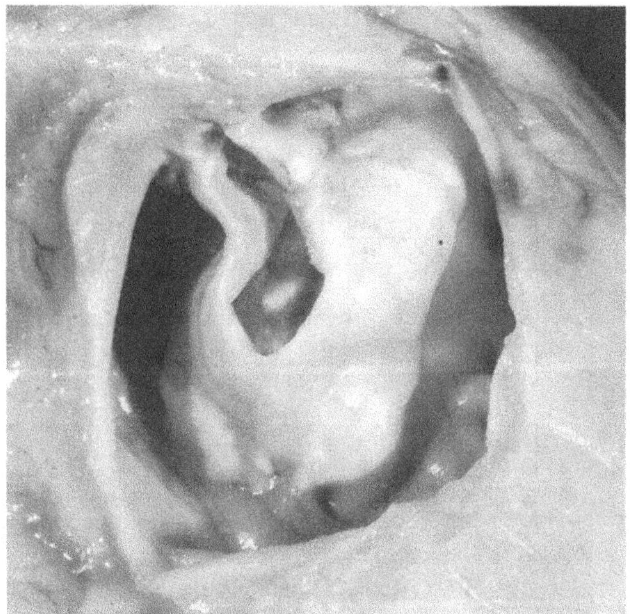

FIGURE 3. Close-up view of the stenotic pulmonic valve from the arterial side.

heavy calcific deposits. The mitral valve had typical anatomic features of prolapse and the valve was incompetent. Both atria were quite dilated and atrial fibrillation was present.

At least 20 patients >40 years of age with unoperated tetralogy of Fallot and studied at necropsy have been reported (Table II).[1–18] In contrast to our patient, none of the 20 patients at necropsy had mitral valve prolapse, and none had a coronary artery anomaly; only 1 survived into the eighth decade, and only 3 had had atrial fibrillation. One (no. 20, Table II) of the 20 patients was reported to have had mitral valve prolapse with severe mitral regurgitation by M-mode echocardiogram, but the mitral prolapse was not confirmed at necropsy.[18]

REFERENCES

1. White PD, Sprague HB. The tetralogy of Fallot. Report of a case in a noted musician who lived to

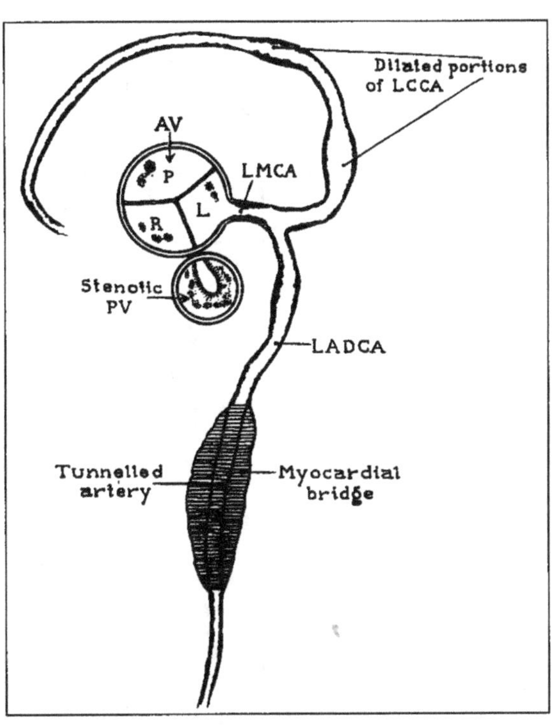

FIGURE 4. Diagram illustrating the origin and course of the coronary arteries. A single coronary ostium is in the left (L) anterior aortic sinus. The left main coronary artery (LMCA) bifurcates into the left circumflex coronary artery (LCCA) and left anterior decending coronary artery (LADCA). The LCCA continues in the left atrioventricular groove to supply the posterior left ventricular wall and right ventricular wall. A portion of the LADCA was tunnelled. The relative sizes of the aortic valve (AV) and the unicuspid, unicommissural, stenotic pulmonic valve (PV) are also shown. P = posterior; R = right.

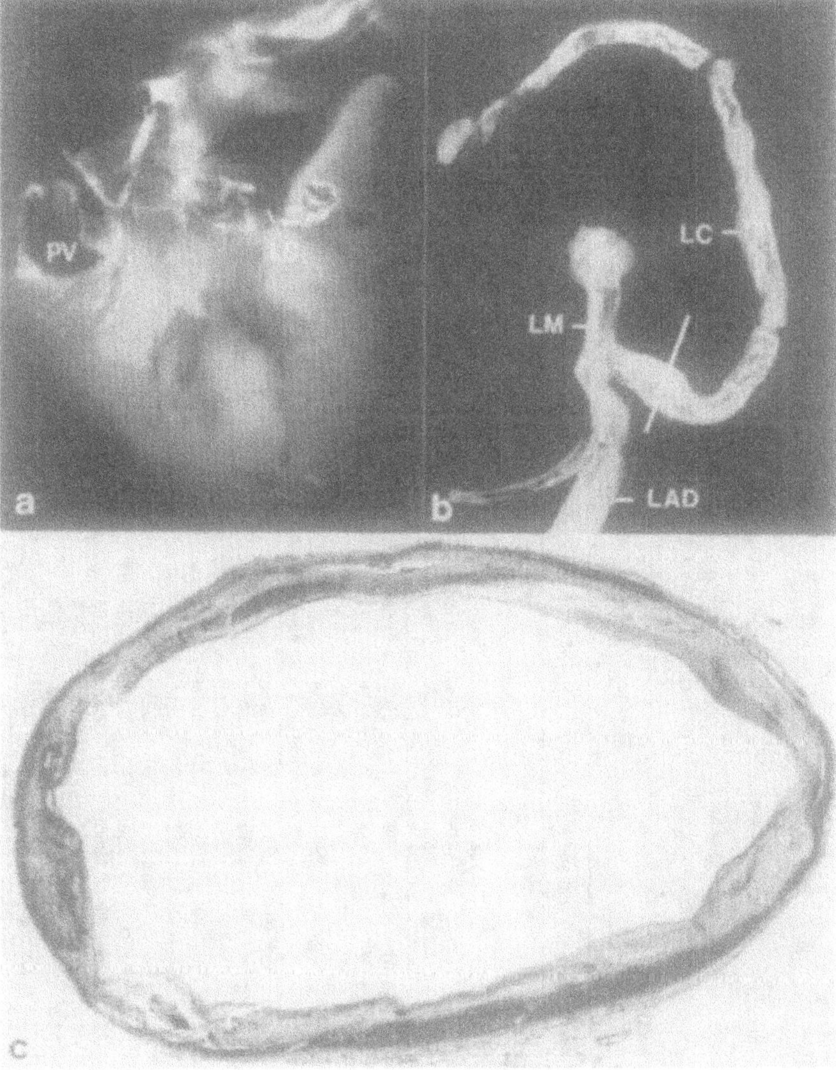

FIGURE 5. Coronary arteries. *a*, radiograph of the intact heart showing calcific deposits in the epicardial coronary arteries, pulmonic valve (PV) and aortic valve. The left circumflex (LC) coronary artery is heavily calcified. *b*, radiograph of the excised coronary arteries showing extensive calcific deposits in the LC coronary artery. *c*, photomicrograph of a section indicated by the *white line in b* of the most dilated portion of the LC coronary artery. (Original magnification ×9, reduced by 27%.) Large calcific plaques are present, but the lumen is widely patent. LM = left main; LAD = left anterior descending.

TABLE II Clinical and Morphologic Features of Previously Published Adults > 40 Years of Age with Unoperated Tetralogy of Fallot and Studied at Necropsy

Case	First Author	Year of Publication	Ref.	Age (yr) at Death & Sex	Age (yr) at Diagnosis	Age (yr) at Onset of CHF	Duration (yr) of CHF	IE by Hx	NYHA FC (1–4+)	BP (s/d)	C	DC	Highest Hgb (g/dl)	Highest Hct (%)	AF	PR Interval (sec)	VA	Mode of Death CHF	Mode of Death CVA	Mode of Death Other	MVP	HW (g)	Site of Outflow Obstruction RV	Site of Outflow Obstruction PV
1	White	1929	1	59M	58	58	1	0	4	110/80	+	+	100%[a]	—	0	0.12	0	0	+	0	0	450	+	0
2	Volini	1938	2	41M	41	35	35	0	3	170/100	+	+	100%[a]	—	0	0.28	0	0	0	+[b]	0	750	+	0
3	Strandell	1939	3	56F	56[c]	—	—	0	4	140/70	+	+	18	—	0	0.17	—	0	0	+[d]	0	370[e]	0	+
4	Feigin	1942	4	53M	37	51	2	0	4	140/70	+	+	98%[a]	—	+	0.24[f]	+	+	0	0	0	970	+	0
5				43F	Birth	25	18	0	4	230/160	+	+	98%[a]	—	0	—	0	+	0	0	0	600	+	0
6	Middleton	1947	5	45M	3	44	1	0	4	—	+	+	21	61	0	0.32	0	+	0	0	0	790	0	+
7	Lian	1949	6	55F	Infancy	—	—	0	3	140/85	+	0	—	—	0	—	+	0	+	0	—	—	+	+
8	Civen	1950	7	47M	27	—	0	—	—	140/80	—	—	—	—	—	—	—	0	0	+[g]	0	650	+	0
9	Baguena	1951	8	44M	44[c]	32	12	0	2	125/65	+	+	120%[a]	—	0	—	—	0	0	+[h]	—	—	0	+
10	Miller	1952	9	56M	Childhood	—	0	0	1	120/85	+	+	23	—	+[i]	0.16[f]	0	0	0	+	0	425	0	+
11	Bain	1954	10	69M	1	67	2	0	4	130/75	+	0	13	—	0	—	+	+	0	0	0	450	+	0
12	Bedford	1956	11	53F	32	48	4	—	3	—	+	–	126%[a]	—	—	—	—	0	+	0	—	480	0	+
13	Rosenthal	1956	12	53F	53[c]	—	0	0	1	170/90	0	0	—	—	0	—	0	0	0	+[g]	—	—	+	0
14	Marquis	1956	13	64F	9	—	0	0	3	150/105	+	+	23	—	0	—	—	0	+	0	—	—	+	+
15				47M	4	—	0	0	1	130/100	+	+	23	—	0	0.12	0	0	0	+[j]	0	—	+	0
16	Abraham	1961	14	48F	19	—	—	0	4	140/90	+	+	—	—	0	—	0	0	0	+[k]	0	450	0	+
17	Bowie	1961	15	68F	Childhood	—	—	0	4	140/80	+	+	18	56	0	0.24	+	0	+	0	0	512	0	+
18	Meindok	1964	16	62M	57	62	0[l]	+	1	170/100	+	0	18	—	0	—	+	0	0	+[m]	—	710	0	+
19	Oakley	1966	17	58M	45	53	5	+	4	115/85	+	+	19	62	+	0.08[f]	+	+	0	0	0	660	+	0
20	Thomas	1987	18	77M	77[c]	73	0	+	1	—	+	+	—[n]	—[n]	0	—	0	+	0	0	0	—	+	0

[a]Hemoglobin measurement as a percentage of a standard based on the method used; [b]chronic glomerulonephritis; [c]diagnosis made at necropsy; [d]tuberculosis; [e]patient weighed 48 kg; [f]measured before onset of atrial fibrillation; [g]cancer; [h]sudden death in hospital unassociated with CHF; [i]complication of bowel surgery; [j]pulmonary infarct; [k]pneumonia; [l]CHF developed with acute myocardial infarction; [m]acute myocardial infarction secondary to atherosclerotic coronary artery disease; [n]"not polycythemic."

AF = atrial fibrillation; BP = blood pressure; C = cyanosis; CHF = congestive heart failure; CVA = cerebrovascular accident; DC = digital clubbing; F = female; FC = functional class; Hct = hematocrit; Hgb = hemoglobin; HW = heart weight; Hx = history; IE = infective endocarditis; M = male; MVP = mitral valve prolapse; NYHA = New York Heart Association; s/d = peak systole/end diastole; PV = pulmonic valve; Ref. = reference; RV = right ventricle; VA = ventricular arrhythmias.

2. Volini IF, Flaxman B. Tetralogy of Fallot. Report of a case in a man who lived to his forty-first year. *JAMA* 1938;111:2000–2003.

3. Strandell B. Fallot's tetrad — fall av sällsynt duration. *Svenska Läkartidningen* 1939;36:1513–1520.

4. Feigin I, Rosenthal J. The tetralogy of Fallot. *Am Heart J* 1943;26:302–312.

5. Middleton WS, Ritchie G. The tetralogy of Fallot. An account of a patient with this condition surviving over forty-five years. *Am Heart J* 1947;33:250–253.

6. Lian C, Fleury J. Survie jusqú á 55 ans d'une maladie bleue (type Fallot). *Arch Mal Coeur* 1949;42:1209–1210.

7. Civin WH, Edwards JE. Pathology of the pulmonary vascular tree. I. A comparison of the intrapulmonary arteries in Eisenmenger complex and in stetricular origin of the aorta. *Circulation* 1950;2:545–551.

8. Báguena R, Tormo V. Coexistencia de tetralogía de Fallot y persistencia del conducto arterioso en una persona de cuarenta y cuatro años. *Med Esp* 1951;26:134–136.

9. Miller SI. Tetralogy of Fallot: report of a case that survived to his fifty-seventh year and died following surgical relief of gall-stone ileus. *Ann Intern Med* 1952;36:901–910.

10. Bain GO. Tetralogy of Fallot: survival to seventieth year. Report of a case. *Arch Pathol* 1954;58:176–179.

11. Bedford DE. Two cases of Fallot's tetralogy, shown at the section in 1929, exhibiting unusual longevity. *Proc R Soc Med* 1956;46:314–315.

12. Rosenthal L. Longevity and the tetralogy of Fal-

13. Marquis RM. Longevity and the early history of the tetralogy of Fallot. *Br Med J* 1956;1:819–822.

14. Abraham AS, Atkinson M, Mitchell WM. Fallot's tetralogy with some features of Marfan's syndrome and survival to 58 years. *Br Heart J* 1961;23:110–112.

15. Bowie EA. Longevity in tetralogy and trilogy of Fallot. Discussion of cases in patients surviving 40 years and presentation of two further cases. *Am Heart J* 1961;62:125–132.

16. Meindok H. Longevity in the tetralogy of Fallot. *Thorax* 1964;19:12–14.

17. Oakley C, Olsen E. A case of long survival with Fallot's tetralogy. *Br Med J* 1966;2:748–753.

18. Thomas SHL, Bass P, Pambakian H, Marigold JH. Cyanotic tetralogy of Fallot in a 77 year old man. *Postgrad Med J* 1987;63:361–362.

Clinical and Morphologic Features of Mitral Valve Prolapse in Octogenarians

Jamshid Shirani, MD,* and William C. Roberts, MD†

The frequency of mitral valve prolapse (MVP) in women decreases progressively from the third to the

From the Pathology Branch, National Heart, Lung, and Blood Institutes, National Institutes of Health, Bethesda, Maryland 20892. Manuscript received February 16, 1993; revised manuscript received and accepted May 20, 1993.

*Present address: Medical College of Virginia, Department of Medicine, Division of Cardiology, Box 128, MCV Station, Richmond, Virginia 23298-0128.

†Present address: Baylor Cardiovascular Institute, Baylor University Medical Center, 3500 Gaston Avenue, Dallas, Texas 75246.

ninth decade of life; in men, in contrast, its frequency remains the same from the third to the ninth decade.[1] Of 264 patients with MVP detected by M-mode echocardiography and reported by Savage and associates,[1] only 4 (1.5%) were aged 80 years or over. A previous clinicopathologic study from this laboratory by Dollar and Roberts[2] included 56 patients aged 16 to 70 years. The present study examines clinical and morphologic findings in 12 octogenarians with MVP at necropsy. Al-

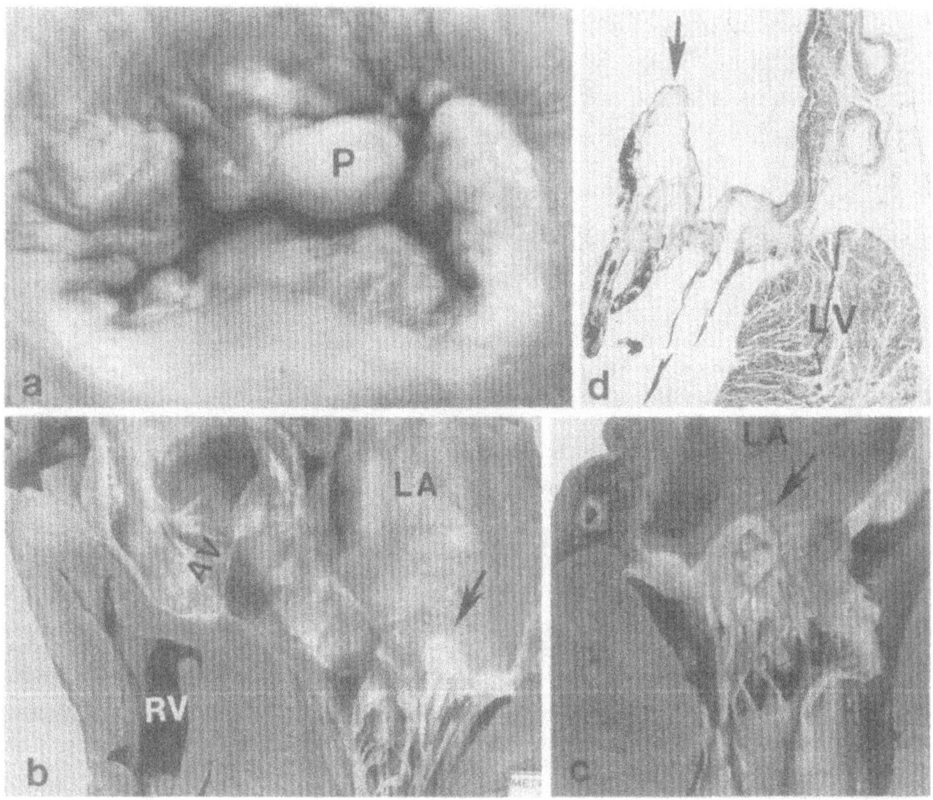

FIGURE 1. The heart of an 80-year-old man (patient 2, GT# 80A-86) who died of gastric lymphoma. On his last hospital admission, a grade 5/6 holosystolic murmur was audible and mitral valve prolapse was diagnosed by echocardiogram. *a,* view of the intact mitral valve from the left atrium (LA) showing prolapsed posterior (P) leaflet. *b,* longitudinal cut showing the posterior one half of the left ventricular outflow tract. The prolapsed portion of posterior mitral leaflet is indicated by the *arrow. c,* longitudinal cut showing the anterior one half of the mitral valve. The arrow again designates the prolapsed portion of the posterior leaflet. *d,* photomicrograph of a histologic section through the prolapsed portion *(arrow)* of the posterior mitral leaflet. The distal two thirds of the leaflet is prolapsed. (Movat stain, original magnification × 2, reduced 35%.) AV = aortic valve; LV = left ventricular wall; RV = right ventricular cavity; VS = ventricular septum.

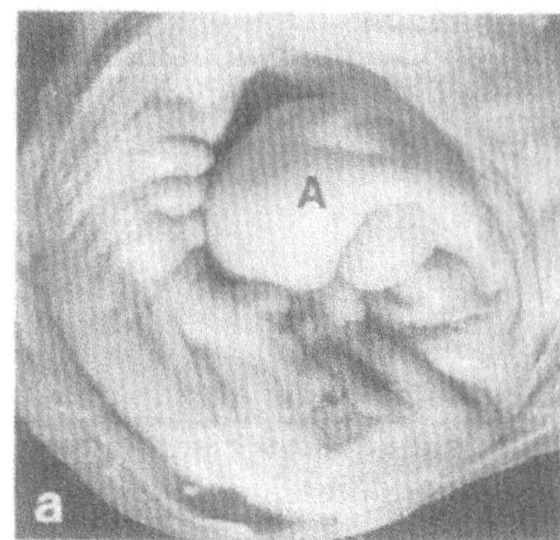
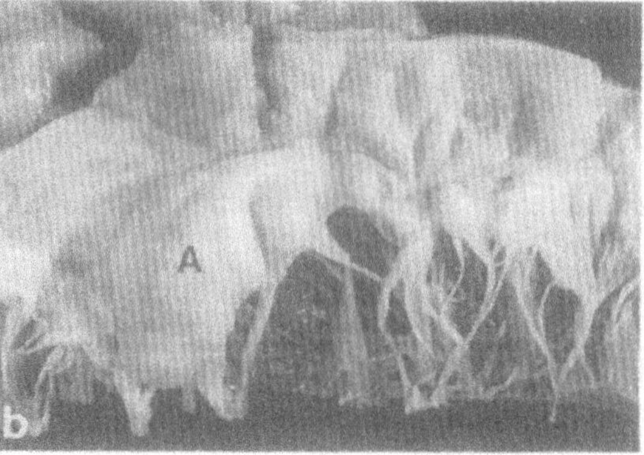

FIGURE 2. The heart of an 81-year-old woman (patient 3, SH #ME-03-1990) who died of pancreatic carcinoma. She never had any signs or symptoms of cardiac dysfunction. On her last admission, a 3/6 holosystolic murmur was heard. *a,* intact mitral valve viewed from the left atrium showing prolapse of the anterior (A) leaflet. *b,* the opened mitral valve showing prominent hooding of the posterior one half of the anterior leaflet.

though patients aged 80 to 89 years have been included in previous necropsy studies of MVP,[3,4] a study focusing exclusively on this age group has not been reported previously.

The necropsy files of the Pathology Branch, National Heart, Lung, and Blood Institute, National Institutes of Health, from January 1956 to February 1993 contain 125 patients coded as having "mitral valve prolapse" or "floppy mitral valve." Twelve of them were 80 to 89 years old at the time of death and are the sub-

TABLE I Certain Clinicopathologic Findings in 12 Octogenarians with Mitral Valve Prolapse

Patient	Age (yr) & Sex	MVP								Cause of Death	HW (g)	LV Fibrosis	Dilated			Chords Missing	Grade of MVP (1-3+)	Plaque Under PML	MVAC (cm)	MAC (0-4+)	VC-PFO	Redundant FO Membrane
		AP	AMI	CHF	SD	SH	Diagnosed Clinically	MR	MVR				RV	LV	CAD							
1	80M	0	0	0	+	0	0	0	0	Sudden death	420	0	0	0	0	0	+++	+	−	0	0	0
2	80M	0	0	+	0	0	+*	+	0	Cancer	415	0	+	0	0	+	+++	0	9.5	0	0	0
3	81F	0	0	0	0	0	0	+	0	Cancer	240	0	0	0	0	+	+++	0	10.5	0	+	0
4	82F	0	0	+	0	+	+†	+	+	Operation‡	360	0	0	0	0	+	+++	0	−	0	0	0
5	82F	0	0	+	0	0	+*	+	0	CHF	390	0	0	+	0	+	+++	0	−	+	0	0
6	82M	+	+	0	0	+	0	0	0	AAA	410	+	0	0	+	0	+	0	9.7	0	0	0
7	82M	0	0	0	0	0	0	0	0	Cancer	460	0	0	0	0	0	++	0	−	0	0	0
8	83M	0	0	+	0	+	0	+	0	Cancer	690	0	0	0	0	0	+	0	12.0	0	0	0
9	84M	+	+	+	0	0	0	+	0	HC§	515	+	0	0	+	+	+++	0	−	+	0	0
10	85F	0	0	+	0	+	0	0	0	Pneumonia	370	0	0	0	0	+	+	+	11.5	++	+	+
11	85F	0	0	+	0	+	0	+	0	IE	330	0	0	0	0	0	++	0	−	0	ASD	0
12	88F	0	0	0	+	0	0	0	0	Car accident	−	0	0	0	0	0	+++	0	−	0	0	0
Totals or (mean)	(83)	2	2	7	2	5	3	7	1		(420)	2	1	1	2	6		2	(10.6)	3	2	1

*Diagnosed by echocardiogram on last hospital admission. †Diagnosed at operation 1 day before death for acute severe mitral regurgitation. ‡Died 1 day after mitral valve replacement. §Not diagnosed during life.

AAA = abdominal aortic aneurysm; AMI = acute myocardial infarction; AP = angina pectoris; ASD = atrial septal defect; CAD = ≥ 1 major epicardial coronary arteries > 75% ↓ in cross-sectional area by plaque; CHF = congestive heart failure; F = female; FO = fossa ovalis; HC = hypertrophic cardiomyopathy; HW = heart weight; IE = infective endocarditis; LV = left ventricle; M = male; MAC = mitral annular calcium; MR = mitral regurgitation; MVAC = mitral valve annular circumference; MVP = mitral valve prolapse; MVR = mitral valve replacement; PML = posterior mitral leaflet; RV = right ventricle; SD = sudden death; SH = systemic hypertension; VC-PFO = valvular-competent patent foramen ovale.

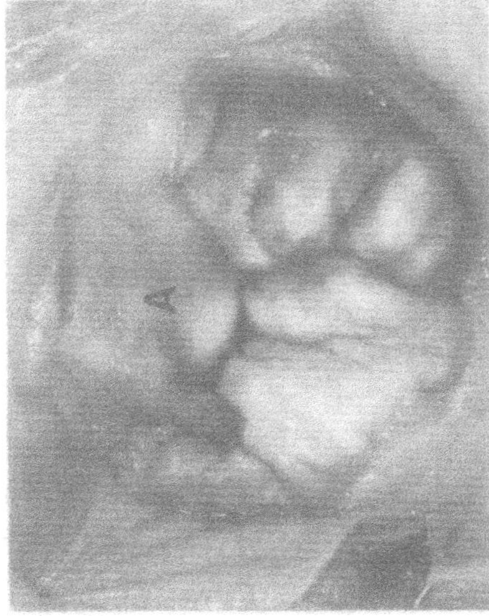

FIGURE 3. View of the intact mitral valve from the left atrium in an 82-year-old man (patient 7, NNMC #A85-127) who died of metastatic adenocarcinoma of the prostate gland. He never had signs or symptoms of cardiac dysfunction. The prolapse involves the posterior leaflet. A = anterior leaflet.

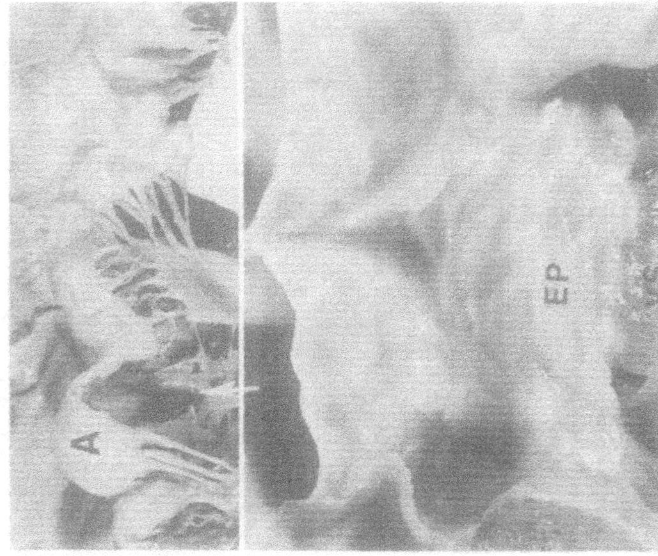

FIGURE 4. The heart of an 84-year-old man (patient 9, WHC #A86-17) with hypertrophic cardiomyopathy. He died during an operation for presumed constrictive pericarditis. *Top,* opened mitral valve showing thickened leaflets with marked hooding of the anterior (A) leaflet and missing chordae tendineae *(arrow). Bottom,* portion of the opened aortic valve and left ventricular outflow tract showing fibrous thickening of the mural endocardium (endocardial plaque). EP = endocardial plaque; VS = ventricular septum.

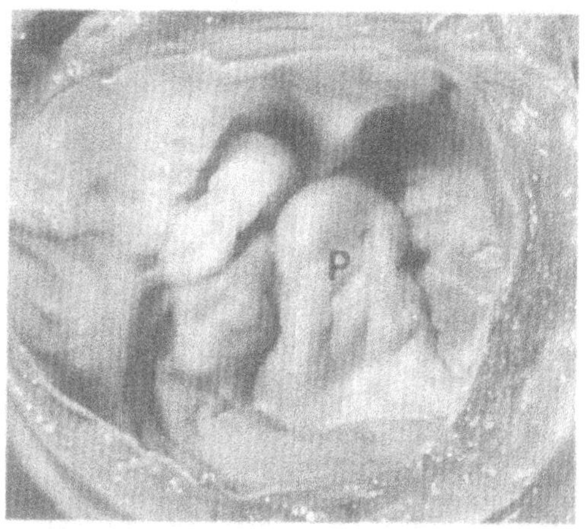

FIGURE 5. Intact mitral valve from left atrium of an 85-year-old woman (patient 10, SH #A87-18) who died of pneumonitis while taking tocainide for symptomatic ventricular tachycardia. Portions of the posterior (P) leaflet are prolapsed. A precordial murmur consistent with mitral regurgitation was audible. Echocardiogram on her last hospital admission did not show mitral prolapse but it did show mitral regurgitation.

jects of this study. They are among 384 patients aged 80 to 89 years at death studied at necropsy in this laboratory.

The following criteria were used to diagnose MVP: (1) the distance from the margin of attachment to distal margin of a portion of posterior mitral leaflet >1.5 cm; and (2) a portion of mitral leaflet protruding into left atrium, i.e., cephalad to the level of the mitral valve annulus.

Certain clinical and morphologic findings in the 12 patients are summarized in Table I and illustrated in Figures 1 to 6. The patients ranged in age from 80 to 88 years (mean 83); 6 were men and 6 were women. Signs and symptoms of congestive heart failure were present in 7 patients, and in 6 of the 7, MVP was the only reasonable cause of the failure. Although a mur-

mur consistent with mitral regurgitation had been heard during life in 7 patients, MVP was diagnosed clinically in only 3 patients (2 by echocardiography during their last hospital admission and 1 at operation for acute severe mitral regurgitation). Death appeared to be related to the MVP in 4 patients (numbers 1, 4, 5 and 11, Table I). At necropsy, the left and right ventricular cavities were of normal size by gross inspection in 11 patients. The mural endocardium behind the posterior mitral leaflet was thickened by fibrous tissue in 2 patients. Calcium was present in the mitral annulus in 3 patients, but its quantity was only mild in each (1–2+/4+). Two patients had a probe-patent valvular-competent foramen ovale which in 1 was associated with redundancy of the fossa ovalis membrane, and 1 patient (number 11) had a secundum atrial septal defect.

Although 7 of the 12 patients in our study had mitral regurgitation by auscultation, and 7 were treated for congestive heart failure, MVP was diagnosed in life in only 3 patients. In all 3, the diagnosis was made during their last hospital admission. Death appeared to be related to the MVP in 4 of the 12 patients. Death was sudden and at home in 1 patient who never had any symptoms or signs of cardiac dysfunction during life, and in whom, except for MVP, no anatomic abnormalities were found at necropsy. Two patients died of congestive heart failure (patients 4 and 5), and a cause other than MVP was not apparent. Death in 1 patient resulted from complications of alpha Streptococcus endocarditis involving the prolapsed mitral valve. In addition to these 4 fatal cases, 2 other patients had congestive heart failure associated with mitral regurgitation. In the remaining 6 patients, MVP caused no cardiac dysfunction and was an incidental finding at necropsy.

This study indicates that MVP may be present in persons aged 80 to 89 years at death, and that the MVP in them may be asymptomatic or cause fatal or nonfatal symptoms of cardiac dysfunction.

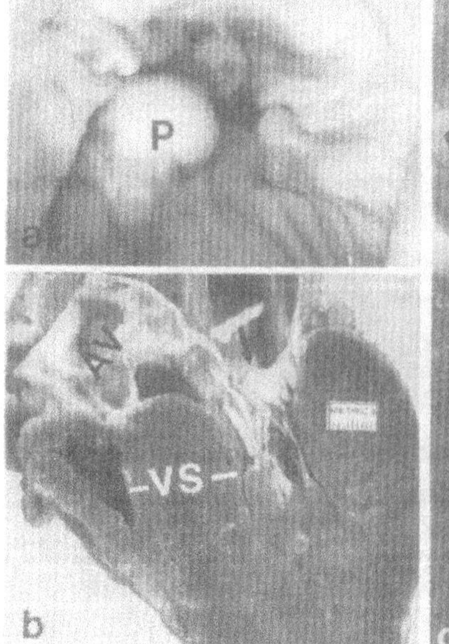

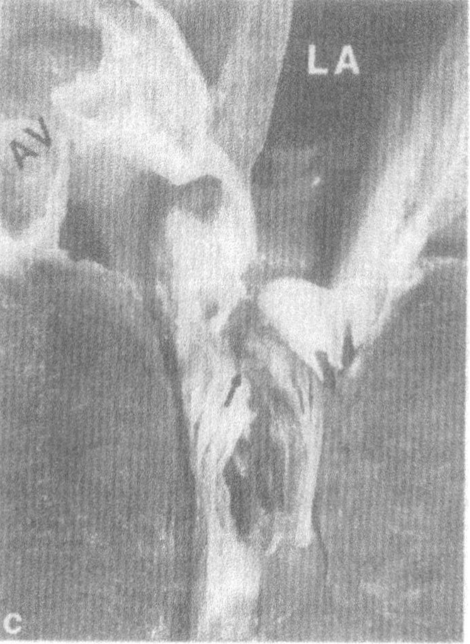

FIGURE 6. Heart of an 85-year-old woman (SH #A84-16) who died of complication of alpha Streptococcus endocarditis involving the prolapsed mitral valve. Mitral valve prolapse was not diagnosed during life. a, view of the intact mitral valve from the left atrium (LA) showing prolapse mainly of the posterior (P) leaflet. b, longitudinal section of the heart showing prolapsed (arrow) posterior mitral leaflet. The left ventricular cavity is small. c, close-up view of the mitral valve showing vegetation (arrow) on the posterior mitral leaflet. AV = aortic valve; VS = ventricular septum.

1. Savage DD, Garrison RJ, Devereux RB, Castelli WP, Anderson SJ, Levy D, McNamara PM, Stokes J, Kannel WB, Feinleib M. Mitral valve prolapse in the general population. I. Epidemiologic features: the Framingham study. *Am Heart J* 1983;106:571–576.

2. Dollar AL, Roberts WC. Morphologic comparison of patients with mitral valve prolapse who died suddenly with patients who died from severe valvular dysfunction or other conditions. *J Am Coll Cardiol* 1991;17:921–931.

3. Pomerance A. Balooning deformity (mucoid degeneration) of atrioventricular valves. *Br Heart J* 1969;31:343–351.

4. Davies MJ, Moore BP, Braimbridge MV. The floppy mitral valve. Study of incidence, pathology, and complications in surgical, necropsy, and forensic material. *Br Heart J* 1978;40:468–481.

Frequency of Atrial Fibrillation in Patients Having Mitral Valve Repair or Replacement for Pure Mitral Regurgitation Secondary to Mitral Valve Prolapse

Rafic Fouad Berbarie, MD[a,b], and William Clifford Roberts, MD[a,b,c,*]

Relatively little attention has been paid to the frequency of atrial fibrillation (AF) in patients with mitral regurgitation (MR) secondary to mitral valve prolapse (MVP). We reviewed clinical, electrocardiographic, echocardiographic, hemodynamic, and angiographic findings in 246 patients aged 21 to 84 years (mean 61) (66% men) who had mitral valve repair or replacement for MR secondary to MVP. Immediately before the mitral operation by electrocardiogram, only 37 patients (15%) had AF and the other 209 patients were in sinus rhythm. Of the latter, 32 had had a history of AF that had reverted to sinus rhythm spontaneously or with antiarrhythmic therapy. Thus, a total of 69 patients (28%) had AF at some time. In conclusion, the frequency of AF in patients with MR secondary to MVP and sick enough to warrant a mitral valve operation have a relatively low frequency of AF (persistent in 15%, paroxysmal in another 13%), percentages considerably lower than that seen in patients with mitral stenosis just before a mitral commissurotomy or replacement. © 2006 Elsevier Inc. All rights reserved. (Am J Cardiol 2006;97:1039–1044)

Since its initial description in 1963, numerous articles on various aspects of mitral valve prolapse (MVP) have appeared.[1] Indeed, from 1966 to 2000, a total of 3,772 articles on MVP were cited on a Medline search. Although many articles mentioned atrial fibrillation (AF), few have focused on its frequency. This report focuses on the frequency of AF in a large group of patients having either mitral valve repair or replacement for mitral regurgitation (MR) secondary to MVP. The hypothesis was that the frequency of AF preoperatively would be relatively small despite the frequency of relatively large atrial cavities.

Methods

From March 1993 to January 2005, a total of 274 patients had mitral valve repair or replacement for pure, i.e., no element of mitral stenosis, MR secondary to MVP at Baylor University Medical Center. All of these operatively excised valves or portions of the valves were examined by 1 of us (WCR), and the etiology of the MR was determined by gross (and often histologic) examination of the operatively excised valve tissue plus examination of the medical record.[2] Of the 274 patients, 28 were eliminated from the present study because of a previous cardiac operation (10

patients), having a pacemaker (5 patients), having a procedure performed simultaneously on the aortic valve (1 patient), or because the clinical chart was unavailable for review (12 patients). The remaining 246 patients were included in the present study. The mitral operation in these patients was their first cardiac operation; all were >20 years of age, none had tricuspid valve replacement, or a procedure performed on the aortic valve.

The electrocardiogram immediately before the mitral operation was reviewed in all 246 patients. Hemodynamic data from cardiac catheterization was available in 143 patients (58%); coronary angiographic data were also available in 217 patients (88%); and echocardiographic data were available in 94 patients (38%).

Statistical analysis was completed using GB-STAT version 10.0 (Dynamic Microsystems Inc., 2004). Variables are expressed as means, with corresponding ranges or frequencies, with corresponding percentages. Means and frequencies were compared with Student's *t* tests. The patients were divided and compared by preoperative rhythm, age, sex, and whether mitral repair or replacement was done. A p value <0.05 was considered statistically significant.

Results

The major findings in the 246 patients are listed in Table 1. The patients were divided into 2 groups: (1) those in whom the electrocardiogram immediately before the mitral valve operation disclosed sinus rhythm (n = 209; 85%); and (2) those in whom the electrocardiogram immediately preoperatively

From the [a]Baylor Heart & Vascular Institute, and the Departments of [b]Medicine (Division of Cardiology) and [c]Pathology, Baylor University Medical Center, Dallas, Texas. Manuscript received October 11, 2005; revised manuscript received and accepted November 4, 2005.

* Corresponding author: Tel: 214-820-7911; fax: 214-820-7533.

E-mail address: wc.roberts@baylorhealth.edu (W.C. Roberts).

Table 1

Preoperative clinical findings in 246 patients with and without pre-op atrial fibrillation by electrocardiogram immediately before mitral valve operation for mitral regurgitation secondary to mitral valve prolapse

Variable	Atrial Fibrillation		p Value
	No (n = 209) (85%)	Yes (n = 37) (15%)	
Age (years): range (mean)	21–81 (59)	34–84 (69)	<0.0001
White	191 (91%)	37 (100%)	<0.06
Men:women	143 (68%):66 (32%)	20 (54%):17 (46%)	0.10
Echocardiographic dimensions (mm) (mean)			
Left atrium	29–65 (50)	41–76 (54)	0.16
Left ventricular peak systole	13–48 (36)	17–50 (38)	0.53
Left ventricular end diastole	18–79 (60)	39–61 (56)	0.22
Pressures (mm Hg) (range) (mean)			
Pulmonary artery peak systole	17–87 (39)	41–76 (44)	0.12
Pulmonary artery mean	10–62 (25)	10–50 (29)	0.15
Left ventricular peak systole	68–198 (125)	89–190 (124)	0.92
Left ventricular end-diastole	3–36 (19)	9–39 (19)	0.99
Pulmonary artery wedge mean	3–43 (17)	5–31 (20)	<0.08
Right ventricular peak systole	12–83 (39)	20–71 (43)	0.14
Right ventricular end-diastole	2–24 (11)	4–25 (12)	0.52
Right atrial mean	1–35 (7)	1–20 (10)	<0.004
Aorta (peak systole)	68–200 (126)	87–199 (126)	0.90/0.67
(end diastole)	39–98 (70)	50–99 (71)	
Other hemodynamic			
Cardiac index (L/min/m^2)	1.4–5.4 (2.7)	1.5–4.1 (2.3)	<0.06
Ejection fraction (%)	30–75 (58)	25–70 (51)	0.0003
Body mass index (kg/m^2)(mean)	26	24	<0.006
≤25	109 (52%)	24 (65%)	0.15
26–30	77 (37%)	12 (32%)	0.56
>30	23 (11%)	1 (3%)	0.13
Systemic hypertension	106 (51%)	20 (54%)	0.74
Mean New York Heart Association functional class (mean)	2.4	2.9	<0.002
I	38 (18%)	3 (8%)	
II	74 (35%)	6 (16%)	<0.002
III	76 (36%)	20 (54%)	
IV	21 (11%)	8 (22%)	<0.002
Number of major coronary arteries narrowed >50% in diameter:	(n = 182)	(n = 35)	
0	139 (77%)	24 (69%)	0.31
1	20 (11%)	3 (9%)	
2	11 (6%)	0 (0%)	
3	8 (4%)	5 (13%)	0.31
Left main	4 (2%)	3 (9%)	
Coronary bypass	42 (20%)	10 (27%)	0.34

disclosed AF (n = 37; 15%). Of the 11 major variables analyzed in the 2 groups, 5 showed significant differences. In contrast to the sinus rhythm group, preoperatively, the AF patients were significantly older (69 vs 59 years), had a lower mean body mass index (24 vs 26 kg/m^2), had a higher New York Heart Association functional class (2.9 vs. 2.4), a higher mean right atrial pressure (10 vs 7 mm Hg), and lower mean ejection fraction (51% vs 58%).

Of the 209 patients with sinus rhythm by electrocardiogram immediately before the mitral valve operation, 32 (15%) had had previous episodes of AF that had either converted to sinus rhythm spontaneously or with use of antiarrhythmic drugs or electrical cardioversion. Thus, of the total 246 patients, 69 (28%) had had ≥1 episode of AF (persistent in 37 and paroxysmal in 32). Comparison of the various variables depicted in Table 1 between the 37 patients with persistent AF and the 32 patients with paroxys-

mal AF disclosed only 1 significant difference: the persistent group had a lower frequency of a history of systemic hypertension than the paroxysmal AF group (20 [54%] vs 23 [72%]; p = 0.01).

Comparison of 12 variables in the men versus the women are presented in Table 2. In contrast to the women, the men had significantly larger left ventricular cavities, lower left ventricular and aortic peak systolic pressures, lower ejection fractions, higher body mass indexes, more angiographic coronary arterial narrowing, and a higher frequency of simultaneous coronary arterial bypass grafting (at the time of the mitral operation).

Comparison of 13 variables in the 157 patients having mitral valve repair versus the 89 patients having mitral valve replacement are listed in Table 3; only 1 significant difference was found—the replacement group had a higher frequency of AF.

Table 2

Comparison of preoperative findings between the men and women who had mitral valve operations for mitral regurgitation secondary to mitral valve prolapse

Variable	Men (n = 163)	Women (n = 83)	p Value
Age (years)	21–84 (60)	27–84 (62)	0.21
White	156 (96%)	72 (87%)	<0.01
AF	20 (12%)	17 (20%)	0.095
Sinus rhythm + history of AF	22 (14%)	10 (12%)	0.66
Sinus rhythm − history of AF	121 (74%)	56 (68%)	0.32
Echocardiographic dimensions (mm)			
Left atrium	29–76 (51)	38–64 (49)	0.52
LV peak systole	13–48 (37)	17–50 (35)	0.36
LV end diastole	18–79 (61)	39–68 (56)	0.03
Pressures (mm Hg) (range)(mean)			
Pulmonary artery peak systole	17–87 (40)	17–86 (40)	0.99
Pulmonary artery mean	10–62 (26)	10–52 (26)	0.85
LV peak systole	68–163 (118)	94–198 (138)	<0.0001
LV end diastole	3–39 (19)	7–36 (18)	0.44
Pulmonary artery wedge mean	3–43 (18)	6–32 (16)	0.31
RV peak systole	12–71 (37)	22–83 (42)	0.05
RV end diastole	2–25 (11)	3–22 (11)	0.47
Right atrial mean	1–20 (7)	1–35 (7)	0.82
Aorta peak systole	68–177 (117)	91–200 (140)	<0.0001
Aorta end diastole	39–90 (67)	47–79 (74)	0.0001
Other hemodynamic data:			
Cardiac index (L/min/m^2)	1.5–5.4 (2.7)	1.5–4.6 (2.7)	0.98
Ejection fraction (%)	25–75 (55)	40–75 (60)	0.0007
Body mass index (kg/m^2) (mean)	26	25	<0.03
≤25	80 (49%)	53 (64%)	<0.03
26–30	65 (40%)	24 (29%)	0.09
>30	18 (11%)	6 (7%)	0.31
Systemic hypertension	79 (48%)	48 (58%)	0.14
Mean NYHA functional class (mean)	2.4	2.5	0.38
I	27 (17%)	14 (17%)	
II	58 (36%)	22 (27%)	0.18
III	60 (36%)	36 (43%)	
IV	18 (11%)	11 (13%)	0.18
No. of major coronary arteries narrowed >50% ↓ in diameter:	(n = 142)	(n = 75)	
0	99 (69%)	65 (80%)	
1	15 (11%)	7 (10%)	<0.004
2	11 (8%)	1 (1%)	
3	12 (8%)	1 (1%)	<0.004
Left main	5 (4%)	1 (1%)	
Coronary bypass	43 (26%)	8 (10%)	<0.004

AF = atrial fibrillation; LV = left ventricular; NYHA = New York Heart Association; RV = right ventricular.

Table 3

Comparison of preoperative findings between patients who had mitral valve repair versus replacement for mitral regurgitation secondary to mitral valve prolapse

Variable	Repair (n = 157)	Replacement (n = 89)	p Value
Age (years)	21–84 (59)	27–84 (62)	0.05
Men	106 (68%)	57 (64%)	0.52
White	147 (94%)	81 (91%)	0.38
AF	18 (11%)	19 (21%)	<0.04
Sinus rhythm + history of AF	26 (17%)	6 (7%)	<0.03
Sinus rhythm − history of AF	113 (72%)	64 (72%)	1.0
Echocardiographic dimensions (mm)			
Left atrium	38–65 (50)	27–76 (51)	0.58
LV peak systole	17–50 (38)	13–48 (34)	0.08
LV end diastole	39–79 (61)	18–79 (57)	0.12
Pressures (mm Hg)			
Pulmonary artery peak systole	17–77 (39)	18–87 (42)	0.15
Pulmonary artery mean	10–50 (25)	10–62 (27)	0.23
LV peak systole	94–83 (125)	68–198 (125)	0.83
LV end-systole	7–36 (19)	3–39 (18)	0.21
Pulmonary artery wedge mean	5–43 (17)	3–32 (18)	0.30
RV peak systole	12–71 (38)	22–83 (42)	0.13
RV end-diastole	3–25 (11)	2–22 (11)	0.79
Right atrial mean	1–35 (7)	1–20 (8)	0.36
Aorta peak systole	87–177 (126)	68–200 (125)	0.94
Aorta end diastole	39–97 (70)	49–99 (70)	0.98
Other hemodynamic data:			
Cardiac index (L/min/m^2)	1.4–4.7 (2.7)	1.5–5.4 (2.6)	0.80
Ejection fraction (%)	25–75 (57)	30–75 (57)	0.87
Body mass index (kg/m^2) (mean)	26	25	0.28
≤25	82 (52%)	50 (56%)	0.54
26–30	60 (38%)	30 (34%)	0.53
<30	15 (10%)	9 (10%)	1
Systemic hypertension	74 (47%)	53 (60%)	0.05
Mean NYHA functional class (mean)	2.4	2.5	0.45
I	26 (17%)	15 (17%)	
II	56 (36%)	24 (27%)	0.18
III	57 (36%)	39 (44%)	
IV	18 (11%)	11 (12%)	0.18
Major coronary arteries narrowed >50% ↓ in diameter:			
0	113/142 (79%)	54/75 (71%)	
1	14/142 (10%)	7/75 (9%)	0.19
2	7/142 (5%)	4/75 (5%)	
3	7/142 (5%)	6/75 (8%)	0.19
Left main	1/142 (1%)	5/75 (7%)	
Coronary bypass	27 (17%)	24 (27%)	0.06

Abbreviations as in Table 2.

Comparison of 13 variables in 3 different age groups (21 to 50 vs 51 to 70 vs >70 years) are listed in Table 4. In comparison to 1 or both of the younger age groups, the 59 patients >70 years of age had a higher frequency of AF, a higher percentage had mitral replacement (compared with repair), higher peak systolic and mean pulmonary arterial pressures, higher left ventricular peak systolic pressures, higher mean pulmonary arterial wedge pressures, higher right ventricular peak systolic pressures, higher peak systolic aortic pressures, lower cardiac indexes, higher New

Table 4
Comparison of the findings by age in patients undergoing mitral valve operation for mitral regurgitation secondary to mitral valve prolapse

Variable	Age Groups (years)			p Values		
	21–50 (n = 57)	51–70 (n = 130)	>70 (n = 59)	1 vs 2	2 vs 3	1 vs 3
Men:women	40 (70%):17 (30%)	89 (68%):41 (32%)	34 (58%):25 (42%)	0.79	0.18	0.18
White	51 (89%)	120 (92%)	57 (97%)	0.51	0.20	<0.10
AF	3 (5%)	12 (9%)	22 (37%)	0.35	0.0001	0.0001
Sinus rhythm (ECG) + history of AF	3 (5%)	24 (18%)	5 (8%)	<0.02	<0.08	0.51
Sinus rhythm (ECG) − history of AF	51 (90%)	94 (72%)	32 (55%)	<0.01	<0.03	0.001
Mitral repair/replacement	40 (70%)/17 (30%)	88 (68%)/42 (32%)	29 (49%)/30 (51%)	0.79	<0.02	<0.03
Echocardiographic dimension (mm):						
Left atrium	39–63 (48)	29–65 (50)	34–76 (51)	0.24	0.92	0.32
LV peak systole	36–47 (40)	13–48 (36)	17–50 (35)	0.18	0.74	<0.07
LV end diastole	56–78 (64)	18–79 (59)	39–73 (57)	0.13	0.39	<0.008
Pressures (mm Hg)						
Pulmonary artery peak systole	17–61 (31)	17–18 (41)	21–86 (44)	<0.002	0.25	0.0001
Pulmonary artery mean	10–44 (21)	10–62 (26)	14–52 (28)	<0.02	0.27	0.0005
LV peak systole	76–167 (118)	68–183 (121)	89–198 (137)	0.50	<0.002	<0.003
LV end-diastole	7–30 (17)	3–39 (19)	7–32 (18)	0.26	0.41	0.70
Pulmonary artery wedge mean	5–28 (13)	3–43 (18)	6–31 (19)	<0.02	0.61	<0.003
RV peak systole	20–66 (33)	20–83 (39)	12–81 (43)	<0.04	0.18	<0.005
RV end-diastole	2–24 (11)	3–22 (11)	3–25 (12)	0.75	0.30	0.62
Right atrial mean	1–12 (6)	1–35 (7)	1–20 (8)	0.30	0.20	<0.03
Aorta peak systole	91–163 (119)	68–177 (122)	87–200 (137)	0.61	<0.002	<0.004
Aorta end-diastole	52–98 (73)	47–94 (69)	39–99 (69)	<0.07	0.84	0.20
Other hemodynamic data:						
Cardiac index (L/min/m^2)	1.9–4.7 (3.0)	1.4–4.3 (2.6)	1.5–5.4 (2.5)	<0.05	0.51	<0.04
Ejection fraction (%)	30–70 (57)	35–75 (58)	25–75 (56)	0.91	0.25	0.47
Body mass index (kg/m^2)	20–41 (25)	17–46 (26)	18–34 (24)	0.11	<0.02	0.50
Systemic hypertension	18 (32%)	71 (55%)	37 (65%)	<0.005	0.20	0.0006
Mean NYHA functional class	2.1	2.4	2.8	<0.02	<0.02	0.0001
I	16 (30%)	19 (15%)	5 (8%)			
II	21 (37%)	46 (35%)	13 (22%)	<0.04	<0.02	0.0001
III	15 (26%)	51 (39%)	30 (51%)			
IV	4 (7%)	14 (11%)	11 (19%)	<0.04	<0.02	0.0001
No. of major coronary arteries narrowed >50% in diameter:	(n = 43)	(n = 120)	(n = 54)			
0	37 (86%)	93 (77%)	34 (63%)	0.21	<0.06	<0.02
1	3 (7%)	13 (11%)	6 (11%)			
2	1 (2%)	8 (7%)	3 (6%)			
3	2 (5%)	5 (4%)	6 (11%)			
Left main	0 (0%)	1 (1%)	5 (9%)			
Coronary bypass	5 (9%)	28 (22%)	18 (31%)	<0.04	0.19	<0.004

ECG = electrocardiogram; other abbreviations as in Table 2.

York Heart Association functional classes, and greater coronary arterial narrowing.

Discussion

The heretofore described data in 246 patients having mitral valve repair or replacement for MR due to MVP disclosed that the frequency of AF preoperatively was relatively low, namely, 15%. Compared with the 209 patients with sinus rhythm preoperatively, the 37 patients with AF were significantly older, less likely to be men, more likely to be lean, more likely to have severe heart failure, to have higher right atrial pressures and lower left ventricular ejection fractions. The frequency of AF in previously published reports of patients with MVP is listed in Table 5.[2–13]

The frequency of AF among patients with MR from MVP severe enough to warrant a mitral operation might logically be expected to be >15% because the disease process would appear to be in a relatively late stage. Earlier stages of MVP, for example, in cases picked up by community screening programs (auscultation, echocardiography) among asymptomatic MVP patients or early symptomatic patients, have an even lower frequency of MVP. Indeed, Freed and colleagues[10] reviewed echocardiograms in 3491 offspring cohorts of the Framingham Heart Study, and found 84 subjects (2.4%) to have MVP. Only 1 (1.2%) had AF. The subjects with MVP were leaner than the subjects without MVP. None had a mitral valve operation. Grigioni and associates[12] analyzed 360 patients (aged 65 ± 13 years; 74% men in the local Rochester, Minnesota, community)

Table 5

Previous publications of patients with mitral valve prolapse showing frequency of atrial fibrillation and other variables

First Author	Year of Publication	Method of Diagnosis of MVP	No. of Patients With MVP	Age (years) Range (mean)	Men	AF	Angiographic Coronary Disease	Mitral Valve Operation
Waller[2]	1982	Surgical	60	36–73 (55)	29 (48%)	4 (7%)	3/23 (13%)	69 (100%)
Ranganathan[3]	1973	S or Autopsy	16	37–69 (—)	9 (56%)	11 (69%)	—	Most
Higgins[4]	1976	Echo	40*	50–90 (65)	40* (100%)	14 (35%)	—	—
Kolibash[5]	1983	Au, Echo, An	62	60–81 (—)	25 (40%)	13 (21%)	4/26 (15%)	21 (34%)
Tresch[6]	1985	Operation	30	25–72 (60)	20 (67%)	13 (43%)	3/29 (10%)	30 (100%)
Penkoske[7]	1985	Operation	31	— (63)	17 (55%)	18 (58%)	9 (29%)	31[†] (100%)
Kolibash[8]	1986	Operation	86	26–82 (60)	53 (62%)	48 (56%)	8 (9%)	76 (88%)
Naggar[9]	1986	Echo	145	≥60	71 (49%)	27 (18%)	—	22 (15%)
Freed[10]	1999	Echo	84[‡]	26–84 (56)	34 (41%)	1 (1%)	—	1 (1%)
Ohki[11]	2001	Echo	118	32–68 (50)	69 (58%)	29 (25%)	—	—
Grigioni[12]	2002	Echo	89[§]	52–78 (65)	59 (66%)	19 (21%)	—	35 (39%)
Avierinos[13]	2002	Echo	833[‖]	29–71 (50)	300 (36%)	67 (8%)	—	65 (8%)

* Studied at a Veterans-Administration Hospital.

[†] Mitral-valve repair in each.

[‡] Diagnosed from a general population survey (Framingham).

[§] Focused on patients with sinus rhythm at diagnosis of "degenerative" mitral regurgitation and percent who developed AF at 5 and 10 years of follow-up.

[‖] Focused on patients with asymptomatic MVP in a community (Rochester).

An = angiography; Au = auscultation; MVP = mitral valve prolapse; S = surgery; other abbreviation as in Table 2.

with MR due to flail mitral leaflet (n = 360) and patients with grade 3 or 4 MR secondary to MVP (n = 89). All 449 patients were in sinus rhythm at diagnosis. By 10 years after diagnosis, however, nearly 50% had developed AF. The patients who developed AF were older and had larger left atria than did those who remained in sinus rhythm.

It is well known that MVP tends to be more frequent in women than in men. It has been estimated that MVP is present in about 8 million adults in the USA. The MVP patients who develop enough MR to warrant mitral valve operation, however, are more often men than women. In the present study, 163 (66%) of the 246 patients were men. The reason for the dominance of men in this circumstance is unclear.

The ages of the patients included in the present study ranged from 21 to 84 years (mean 61). The mean age of these patients places them, of course, in a category where coronary artery disease is relatively frequent. Surprisingly, however, only 54 (22%) had angiographic evidence of narrowing >50% in diameter of ≥1 epicardial coronary artery. A possible explanation for this relatively low frequency of angiographically demonstrated coronary arterial narrowing may be the relatively high frequency of body mass indexes of ≤25 kg/m^2. Of the 246 patients, 134 (54%) had this relatively low body mass index and, furthermore, only 24 (10%) were obese (body mass index >30 kg/m^2).

Why AF appears to be less frequent in adults with MR from MVP than in similar aged adults with mitral stenosis has received virtually no attention. Mitral stenosis in adults is virtually always of rheumatic origin, a process which affects the left atrial wall as well as the mitral valve with or without involvement of other valves.[14] In contrast, MVP has no direct effect on the atrial walls other than the secondary hemodynamic consequences. In other words, the atrial walls are histologically abnormal in patients with mitral stenosis, whereas these walls are histologically normal, except for myofiber hypertrophy, in patients with MVP.

Like virtually all clinical investigations, this work has limitations. An important one is the lack of hemodynamic, angiographic, and echocardiographic data on all the patients included. Another limitation is almost certainly different standards regarding need for operative intervention among the multiple cardiologists referring these patients for cardiac operations. Additionally, some of the cardiac surgeons leaned more to mitral repair versus mitral replacement than did others.

1. Barlow JB, Pocock WA, Marchand P, Denny M. The significance of late systolic murmurs. Am Heart J 1963;66:443–452.
2. Waller BF, Morrow AG, Maron BJ, Del Negro AA, Kent KM, McGrath FJ, Wallace RB, McIntosh CL Roberts WC. Etiology of clinically isolated, severe, chronic, pure mitral regurgitation: analysis of 97 patients over 30 years of age having mitral valve replacement. Am Heart J 1982;104:276–288.
3. Ranganathan N, Silver MD, Robinson TI, Kostuk WJ, Felderhof CH, Patt NL, Wilson JK, Wigle ED. Angiographic-morphologic correlation in patients with severe mitral regurgitation due to prolapse of the posterior mitral valve leaflet. Circulation 1973;48:514–518.
4. Higgins CB, Reinke RT, Gosink BB, Leopold GR. The significance of mitral valve prolapse in middle-aged and elderly men. Am Heart J 1976;91:292–296.
5. Kolibash AJ, Bush CA, Fontana MB, Ryan JM, Kilman J, Wooley CF. Mitral valve prolapse syndrome: analysis of 62 patients aged 60 years and older. Am J Cardiol 1983;52:534–539.
6. Tresch DD, Doyle TP, Boncheck LI, Siegel R, Keelan MH Jr, Olinger GN, Brooks HL. Mitral valve prolapse requiring surgery. Clinical and pathologic study. Am J Med 1985;78:245–250.

7. Penkoske PA, Ellis FH Jr, Alexander S, Watkins E Jr. Results of valve reconstruction for mitral regurgitation secondary to mitral valve prolapse. *Am J Cardiol* 1985;55:735–738.

8. Kolibash AJ Jr, Kilman JW, Bush CA, Ryan JM, Fontana ME, Wooley CF. Evidence for progression from mild to severe mitral regurgitation in mitral valve prolapse. *Am J Cardiol* 1986:58:762–767.

9. Naggar CZ, Pearson WN, Seljan MP, with the technical assistance of Mannock LK, Masrof S, Elwood DJ. Frequency of complications of mitral valve prolapse in subjects aged 60 years and older. *Am J Cardiol* 1986;58:1209–1212.

10. Freed LA, Levy D, Levine RA, Larson MG, Evans JC, Fuller DL, Lehman B, Benjamin EJ. Prevalence and clinical outcome of mitral-valve prolapse. *N Engl J Med* 1999;341:1–7.

11. Ohki R, Yamamoto K, Okayama M, Nonaka M, Suzuki C, Ikeda U, Shimada K. The site of mitral valve prolapse is a predictor of atrial fibrillation. *Am J Cardiol* 2001;88:811–813.

12. Grigioni F, Avierinos J-F, Ling LH, Scott CG, Bailey KR, Tajik AJ, Frye RL, Enriquez-Sarano M. Atrial fibrillation complicating the course of degenerative mitral regurgitation. Determinants of long-term outcome. *J Am Coll Cardiol* 2002;40:84–92.

13. Avierinos J-F, Gersh BJ, Melton LJ III, Bailey KR, Shub C, Nishimura RA, Tajik AJ, Enriquez-Sarano M. Natural history of asymptomatic mitral valve prolapse in the community. *Circulation* 2002;106:1355–1361.

14. Bailey GWH, Braniff BA, Hancock EW, Cohn KE. Relation of left atrial pathology to atrial fibrillation in mitral valve disease. *Ann Intern Med* 1968;69:13–20.

Combined congenitally bicuspid aortic valve and mitral valve prolapse causing pure regurgitation

William C. Roberts, MD, Saleha Zafar, MD, Jong Mi Ko, Melissa M. Carry, MD, and Robert F. Hebeler, MD

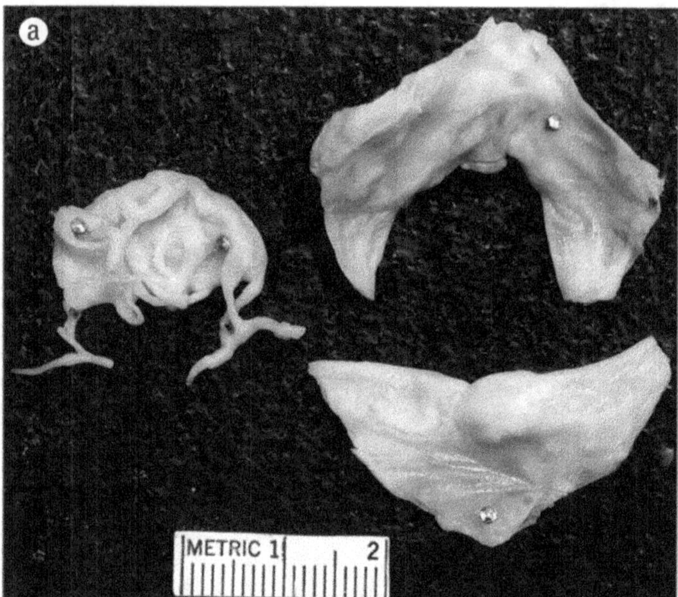

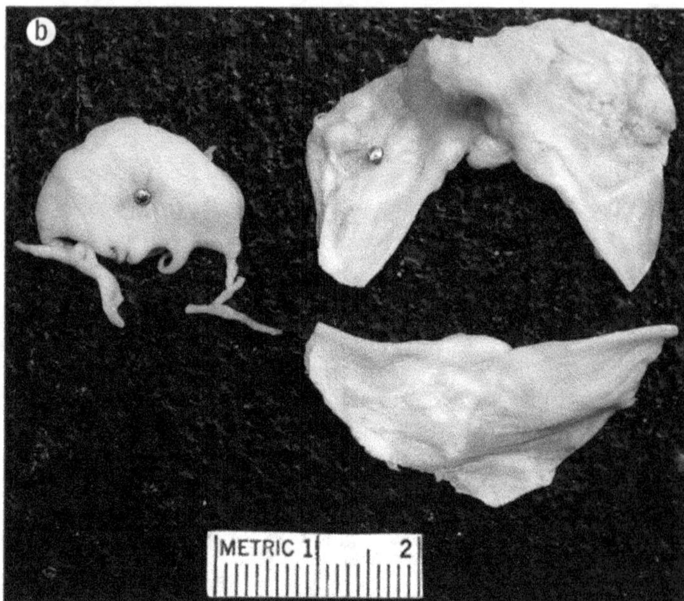

Figure 1. Mitral and aortic valves of the patient described. **(a)** Ventricular aspect of the resected portion of the posterior mitral leaflet and of the congenitally bicuspid aortic valve. Several chordae are missing, indicating that they had ruptured in the past and later became incorporated in the superimposed fibrous tissue on the ventricular aspect of the leaflet (see Figure 2). **(b)** Atrial aspect of the mitral leaflet and aortic aspect of a congenitally bicuspid aortic valve.

Described herein is a patient with a purely regurgitant congenitally bicuspid aortic valve and a purely regurgitant prolapsing mitral valve. Although it is well established that the bicuspid aortic valve is a congenital anomaly, it is less well appreciated that mitral valve prolapse is almost certainly also a congenital anomaly. The two occurring in the same patient provides support that mitral valve prolapse is also a congenital anomaly.

I t is well appreciated that the bicuspid aortic valve (BAV) is usually of congenital origin. It is less well appreciated that mitral valve prolapse (MVP) is usually of congenital origin. Most patients with a congenitally BAV (unless complicated by superimposed infective endocarditis) have a structurally normal mitral valve. It is most unusual for a patient with a congenitally BAV, particularly one that is purely regurgitant, to have associated MVP. Such was the case, however, in the patient described herein.

CASE DESCRIPTION

A 64-year-old white man with a doctorate, who was born in June 1947, had been well until November 2011, when he had the first of several episodes of syncope. During hospitalization for acute appendicitis, an electrocardiogram disclosed the presence of atrial fibrillation. Another syncopal episode and the appearance of exertional and nocturnal dyspnea in 2012 prompted a visit to a cardiologist. His body mass index was 30 kg/m². A grade 2/6 basal precordial systolic murmur and a grade 4/6 blowing apical systolic murmur with radiation into the left axilla were heard. The initial electrocardiogram showed supraventricular tachycardia with a ventricular rate of

From the Divison of Cardiology, Department of Internal Medicine (Roberts, Zafar, Ko, Carry), and Department of Cardiothoracic Surgery (Hebeler), Baylor Heart and Vascular Hospital and Baylor University Medical Center at Dallas.

Corresponding author: William C. Roberts, MD, Baylor Heart and Vascular Institute, 621 North Hall Street, Dallas, TX 75226 (e-mail: wc.roberts@baylorhealth.edu).

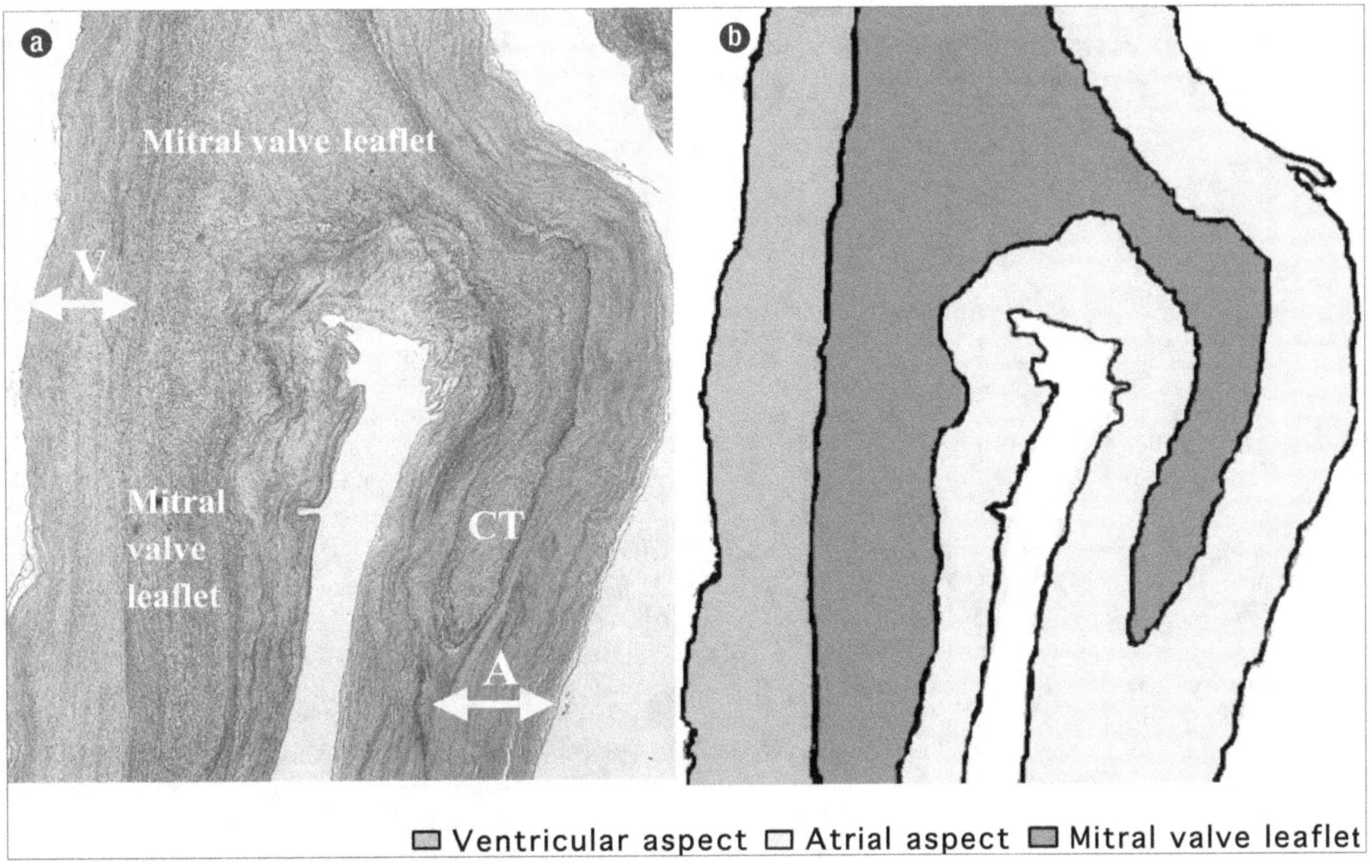

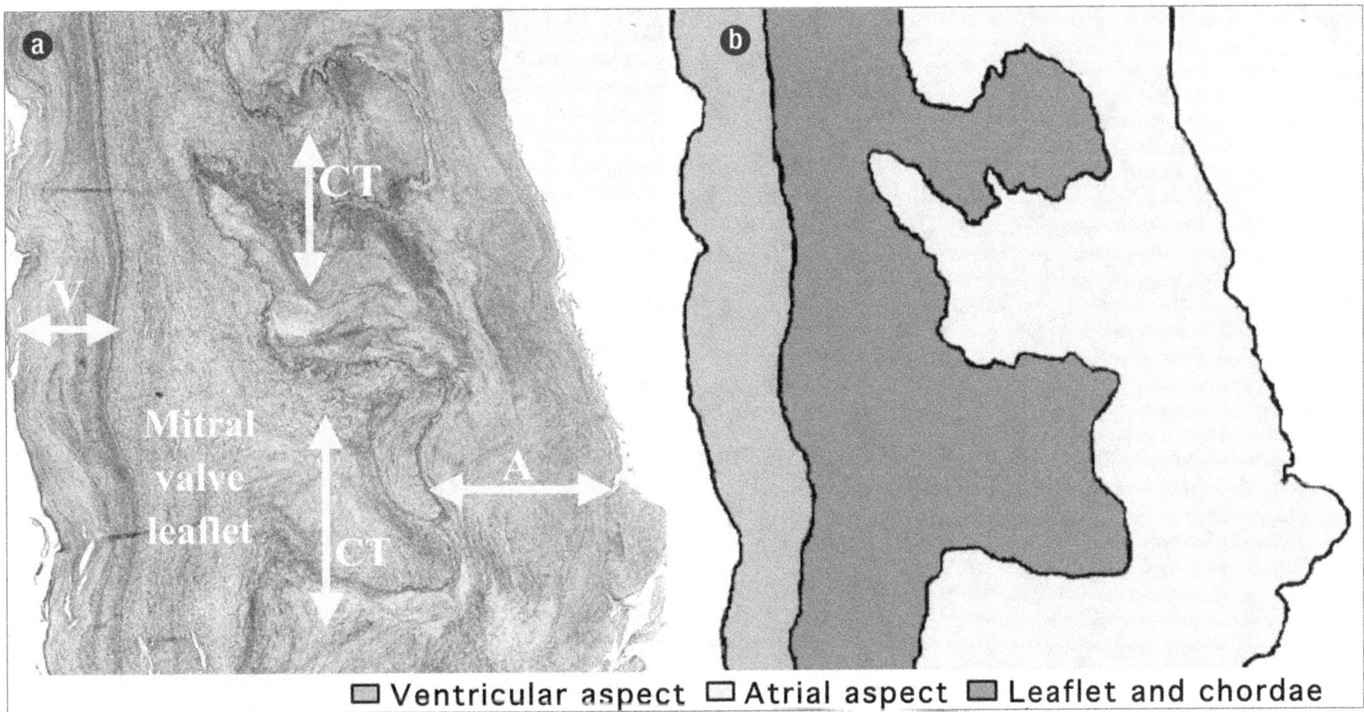

Figure 2. (a) Photomicrograph of a portion of the posterior mitral valve leaflet and attached chordae tendineae (CT). The leaflet and chordal thickening is the result of superimposed fibrous tissue on both atrial (A) and ventricular (V) aspects of the leaflet and surrounding the chordae. The leaflet itself consists primarily of the fibrosa element; the spongiosa element is minimal. These histological features are characteristic of mitral valve prolapse. Elastic von Gieson stain, ×40. **(b)** A color-coded replica with green representing the ventricular aspect, yellow representing the atrial aspect, and red representing the mitral valve leaflet.

Figure 3. (a) Photomicrograph of a portion of the mitral leaflet and chordae tendineae (CT) with superimposed fibrous tissue on the atrial (A) aspect and on the ventricular (V) aspect. The underlying normal leaflet and chordae tendineae are outlined by a black-staining elastic membrane. It is likely that the chordae had ruptured in the distant past and later the portion closest to the leaflet was covered by fibrous tissue. Elastic von Gieson stain, ×40. **(b)** A color-coded replica with green representing the ventricular aspect, yellow representing the atrial aspect, and red representing the leaflet and chordae.

Table. Previously reported patients having simultaneous aortic and mitral valve operations for a dysfunctioning congenitally bicuspid aortic valve and a dysfunctioning mitral valve*

Valve dysfunction	Patients (n)	Ages, years: Range (mean)	Etiology of MR				
			IE	IC	RHD	MVP	Unknown
AS + MS	6	46–74 (59)	0	0	4	0	2
AS + MR	13	52–84 (66)	2	2	0	4	5
AR + MS	0	0	0	0	0	0	0
AR + MR	9	24–66 (46)	7	0	0	1	1
Totals	28	24–84 (56)	9	2	4	5	8

*From Fernicola and Roberts, 1994 (3) and Roberts et al, 2012 (4).
AR indicates aortic regurgitation; AS, aortic stenosis; IC, ischemic cardiomyopathy; IE, infective endocarditis; MR, mitral regurgitation; MS, mitral stenosis; MVP, mitral valve prolapse; RHD, rheumatic heart disease.

140 beats a minute. An echocardiogram showed MVP with a flail P_2 portion of the posterior leaflet and severe mitral regurgitation. The aortic valve was bicuspid, and moderate aortic regurgitation was present. The left ventricular cavity was of normal size, and its ejection fraction was 60%. Cardiac catheterization disclosed the following pressures in mm Hg: left ventricle, 136/33; aorta, 139/70; pulmonary artery wedge, a wave 23, v 38, mean 11; pulmonary artery, 34/13; right ventricle, 39/14; and right atrium, a wave 14, v wave 13, mean 11. The cardiac index was 2.9 L/min/m². Coronary angiogram disclosed no luminal narrowing; the right coronary was the dominant artery. Left ventricular cavity size and contractility were normal. The aortic regurgitation was graded 2+/4+.

Five days later the purely regurgitant aortic valve was replaced with a #29 Mosaic porcine xenograft. The mitral valve was repaired by resecting P_2, replacing two chordae, and inserting a #37 ATS annuloplasty ring *(Figures 1–3)*. Additionally, a Maze procedure was performed. Seven days postoperatively, because of the development of complete atrioventricular disassociation, a dual-chamber pacemaker was inserted. Electrocardiogram in July 2012 disclosed sinus rhythm (75 beats a minute) and complete left bundle branch block. When seen on September 11, 2012, 3 months after the valve operation, the patient was asymptomatic and "feeling great."

DISCUSSION

The occurrence of both a congenitally BAV and MVP in the same patient suggests that both conditions are of congenital origin. That the BAV is a congenital anomaly is well accepted, but that MVP is also likely a congenital anomaly—at least some of the leaflet and chordal tissue is congenitally deficient—is less well appreciated.

Iqbal and colleagues (1) in 1980 appear to have been the first to report MVP associated with a congenital BAV. They described two patients, one a 39-year-old man who underwent mitral and aortic valve replacement for combined mitral and aortic regurgitation and the other, a 23-year-old man with mitral regurgitation and a normally functioning congenitally BAV.

Chisholm (2) in 1981 found a congenitally BAV in 8 of 257 black patients with MVP. None of his 8 patients had either mitral or aortic dysfunction severe enough to warrant operative intervention. All 8 patients had evidence of trace aortic regurgitation, and none had evidence of aortic stenosis. None apparently had significant mitral regurgitation. The cardiac size in all 8 patients was normal.

In 1994 Fernicola and Roberts (3) described 11 patients who underwent aortic valve replacement for a dysfunctioning congenitally BAV and mitral replacement for a purely regurgitant mitral valve. In 2012 Roberts and colleagues (4) described another 16 patients at another institution who had aortic valve replacement for a dysfunctioning congenitally BAV and simultaneous mitral valve operation for a dysfunctioning mitral valve. The *Table* summarizes the findings in the combined studies by Fernicola and Roberts (3) and by Roberts et al (4). Of their 28 patients, the BAV was stenotic in 19 (68%) and purely regurgitant in 9 (32%); the mitral valve was stenotic in 6 (21%) and purely regurgitant in 22 (79%). Of the 19 patients with stenotic BAVs, at least 4 (21%) had MVP; of the 9 patients with a purely regurgitant BAV, only 1 (11%) had MVP, as did the patient described herein.

1. Iqbal MZ, Eybel CE, Messer JV. Mitral valve prolapse associated with bicuspid aortic valve. *Cardiovasc Rev Rep* 1980;1:465–468.
2. Chisholm JC. Mitral valve prolapse syndrome associated with congenital bicuspid aortic valve. *J Natl Med Assoc* 1981;73(10):921–923.
3. Fernicola DJ, Roberts WC. Pure mitral regurgitation associated with a malfunctioning congenitally bicuspid aortic valve necessitating combined mitral and aortic valve replacement. *Am J Cardiol* 1994;74(6):619–624.
4. Roberts WC, Janning KG, Vowels TJ, Ko JM, Hamman BL, Hebeler RF Jr. Presence of a congenitally bicuspid aortic valve among patients having combined mitral and aortic valve replacement. *Am J Cardiol* 2012;109(2):263–271.

Gross and Histological Features of Excised Portions of Posterior Mitral Leaflet in Patients Having Operative Repair of Mitral Valve Prolapse and Comments on the Concept of Missing (= Ruptured) Chordae Tendineae

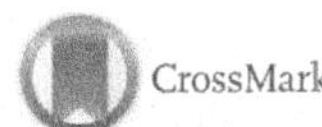

William C. Roberts, MD,*†‡ Travis J. Vowels, BBA,* Jong M. Ko, BA,* Robert F. Hebeler, Jr, MD§

Dallas, Texas

Objectives	The aim of the study is to describe gross and histological features of operatively excised portions of mitral valves in patients with mitral valve prolapse (MVP).
Background	Although numerous articles on MVP (myxomatous or myxoid degeneration, billowing or floppy mitral valve) have appeared, 2 virtually constant histological features have been underemphasized or overlooked: 1) the presence of superimposed fibrous tissue on both surfaces of the leaflets and surrounding many chordae tendineae; and 2) the absence of many chordae tendineae on the ventricular surfaces of the leaflets as the result of their being hidden (i.e., covered up) by the superimposed fibrous tissue.
Methods	We examined operatively excised portions of prolapsed posterior mitral leaflets in 37 patients having operative repair.
Results	Histological study of elastic-tissue stained sections disclosed that the leaflet thickening was primarily due to the superimposed fibrous tissue. All leaflets had variable increases in the spongiosa element within the leaflet itself with some disruption and/or loss of the fibrosa element and occasionally complete separation of it from the spongiosa element. Both the leaflet and chordae were separated from the superimposed fibrous tissue by their black-staining elastic membranes.
Conclusions	These findings demonstrate that the posterior leaflet thickening in MVP is mainly due to the superimposed fibrous tissue rather than to an increased volume of the spongiosa element of the leaflet itself. The superimposed fibrous tissue on both leaflet and chordae is likely the result of subsequent abnormal contact of the leaflets and chordae with one another. Chordal rupture (i.e., missing chordae) occurred in all 37 patients, but finding individual ruptured chords was rare. (J Am Coll Cardiol 2014;63:1667–74) © 2014 by the American College of Cardiology Foundation

Although numerous publications have appeared describing auscultory, angiographic, echocardiographic, and morphological features of mitral valve prolapse (MVP) (myxomatous or myxoid degeneration), surprisingly, none have reproduced the various histological features of the operatively excised

mitral valves or parts thereof in color after staining for elastic fibers, an absolute necessity for proper evaluation, because a black-staining elastic membrane separates the leaflet and chordae from the superimposed fibrous tissue, a constant feature of MVP. In this report, we focus on the contribution of the superimposed fibrous tissue to the leaflet and chordal thickening, and second, we introduce the concept that missing or hidden chords (those lying beneath the superimposed fibrous tissue) are equivalent to ruptured chords.

Methods

Since March 1993, all specimens excised at operation by cardiac surgeons at Baylor University Medical Center at

From the *Baylor Heart and Vascular Institute, Baylor University Medical Center, Dallas, Texas; †Department of Internal Medicine (Division of Cardiology), Baylor University Medical Center, Dallas, Texas; ‡Department of Pathology, Baylor University Medical Center, Dallas, Texas; and the §Department of Cardiothoracic Surgery, Baylor University Medical Center, Dallas, Texas. The study was funded by the Baylor Health Care System Foundation, Dallas, Texas. The authors have reported that they have no relationships relevant to the contents of this paper to disclose.

Manuscript received August 31, 2013; revised manuscript received November 7, 2013, accepted November 12, 2013.

Dallas have been submitted to the surgical pathology division of the pathology department, and all such specimens have been described by one of us (W.C.R.) who submitted the pathology report. Most gross specimens were photographed. After describing the submitted specimen, clinical, echocardiographic, and hemodynamic data were retrieved online via the Baylor University Medical Center at the Dallas Electronic Medical Records and the Apollo Cardiovascular Database. A total of 500 mitral valves or portions thereof were received from January 2005 through June 2013 (Fig. 1). Of this number, 140 patients underwent mitral valve repair or replacement for severe mitral regurgitation (MR) secondary to MVP. After excluding those patients where preoperative echocardiograms (n = 71) were not available to us or histological sections of the excised valves were not prepared or retrievable (n = 14) or the patients had chronic renal failure (n = 4), 51 patients were available for study: 14 had mitral valve replacement and were then excluded from the present study; 37 had mitral valve repair, and in each, portions of the posterior leaflet were studied. Sections of the posterior leaflets were cut from the margin of attachment to the free margin and submitted for histological preparation. After processing in alcohol and xylene, 2 sections were cut

from each paraffin block: one was stained by hematoxylin/eosin, and the other, by elastic van Geison.

Results

Pertinent data from the 37 patients are summarized in Table 1. (Data on the 14 patients having mitral valve replacement for MVP are shown in the table simply for comparison.) The operative report in all 37 patients indicated "prolapse" of a portion of posterior mitral leaflet and that the prolapsed segment was the one almost always excised. None of the 37 had calcific deposits in the operatively excised specimens. All 37 patients also had an annular ring inserted.

Examination of the posterior mitral leaflet in the 37 patients disclosed several consistent features (Figs. 2 to 9, Table 2). All 37 operatively excised portions of posterior mitral leaflet had "missing" (i.e., ruptured) chordae tendineae on gross examination. Histologically, the leaflet itself and the chordae tendineae were clearly demarcated by an elastic membrane (elastic van Geison stain). Both atrial and ventricular aspects of the leaflet in all 37 patients contained superimposed fibrous tissue, thicker on the atrial side than on the ventricular side. Additionally, numerous elastic fibers were present in the superimposed fibrous tissue on the atrial aspect, whereas few if any were present in the superimposed fibrous tissue on the

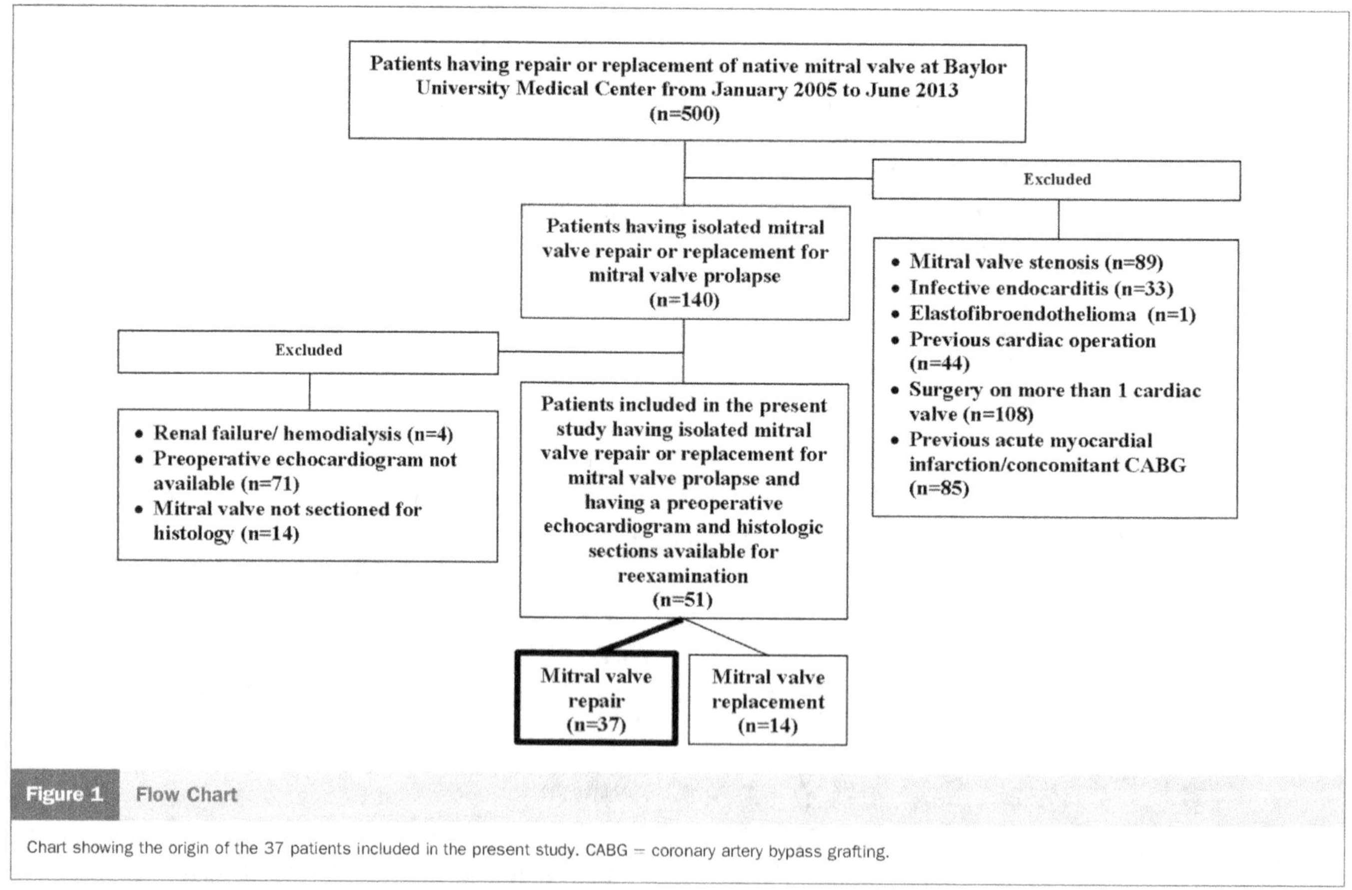

Figure 1   Flow Chart

Chart showing the origin of the 37 patients included in the present study. CABG = coronary artery bypass grafting.

Variable	MV Repair (n = 37) (73%)	MV Replacement* (n = 14) (27%)
Age (yrs)	56 ± 13 [59] (31–78)	59 ± 15 [56] (34–79)
Sex		
M	31 (84%)	7 (50%)
F	6 (16%)	7 (50%)
Ethnicity		
W	32 (86%)	11 (79%)
B	2 (5%)	3 (21%)
H	2 (5%)	0
A	1 (3%)	0
Atrial fibrillation	13 (35%)	7 (50%)
Pressures (mm Hg)		
Pulmonary arterial wedge (n = 29)	15 ± 5 [15] (7–27)	21 ± 10 [21] (6–39)
RV		
Peak systole (n = 32)	39 ± 13 [34] (16–70)	44 ± 15 [41] (18–66)
End diastole (n = 32)	11 ± 4 [11] (2–19)	14 ± 6 [14] (3–23)
Right atrial mean (n = 31)	7 ± 4 [5] (0–16)	11 ± 8 [11] (0–21)
LV		
Peak systole (n = 34)	120 ± 19 [118] (90–162)	115 ± 16 [111] (99–144)
End diastole (n = 36)	18 ± 6 [18] (6–31)	19 ± 8 [16] (12–35)
Aorta		
Peak systole (n = 34)	117 ± 19 [115] (79–147)	121 ± 19 [120] (95–155)
End diastole (n = 34)	66 ± 15 [69] (19–93)	73 ± 15 [69] (56–101)
Cardiac index (l/min/m^2) (n = 27)	2.66 ± 0.48 [2.63] (1.97–3.71)	2.25 ± 0.68 [2.34] (1.38–3.35)
EF (%) (n = 30) (by catheterization)	60 ± 10 [65] (30–75)	55 ± 20 [60] (25–80)
MV regurgitation		
3+	3 (8%)	2 (14%)
4+	34 (92%)	12 (86%)
MV weight (g)	0.70 ± 0.46 [0.51] (0.20–1.94)	1.52 ± 1.18 [1.50] (0.04–4.07)
MV size (mm)		
Ring	31 ± 3	—
Prosthesis	—	29 ± 3

Values are mean ± SD, [median], (range), or n (%). *These cases are included here simply for quick comparison with the patients having mitral valve (MV) repair.

A = Asian; B = black; EF = ejection fraction; H = Hispanic; LV = left ventricle; RV = right ventricle; W = white; + = positive or present; 0 = negative or absent.

ventricular aspect. The fibrous tissue surrounding the chordae tendineae was similar to that on the ventricular aspect of the leaflet. Within the mitral leaflet itself—enclosed by the elastic membrane—the spongiosa element seemed increased in quantity in all patients, more so in the distal one-half than in the proximal one-half of the leaflet; and the fibrosa element was interrupted focally and/or decreased in quantity or both.

Discussion

Examination of operatively excised portions of posterior mitral leaflet in each of the 37 patients having mitral repair for MVP produced 2 major findings: 1) the leaflet and chordal thickening in patients with MVP is due in large part to superimposed fibrous tissue on both the atrial and ventricular surfaces of the leaflets and surrounding the chordae tendineae; and 2) rupture of posterior leaflet chordae tendineae is a nearly universal finding in patients with MVP, and MR is severe enough to warrant operative repair but that seeing 1 or more ruptured chordae is infrequent, because they are covered ("hidden") by the superimposed fibrous tissue on the ventricular surface of the leaflet. In essence, the absence of chordae (missing chordae) is synonymous with earlier rupture of chordae.

We surmise that the superimposed fibrous tissue on both leaflet and chordae is entirely due to abnormal contact of the leaflets with one another over many years or decades. That the underlying leaflet and chordae are essentially intact suggests that the basic process in MVP is a slow, gradual loss and/or interruption of collagen fibers (in the fibrosa element of the leaflet and in the chordae tendineae, which are devoid of a spongiosa element). The loss and/or interruption of collagen fibers within the leaflet and chordae seems to be responsible for the gradual elongation of the leaflets and chordae in MVP, which in turn leads to inappropriate leaflet contact and to the superimposed fibrous tissue ("callus" formation) (Fig. 10).

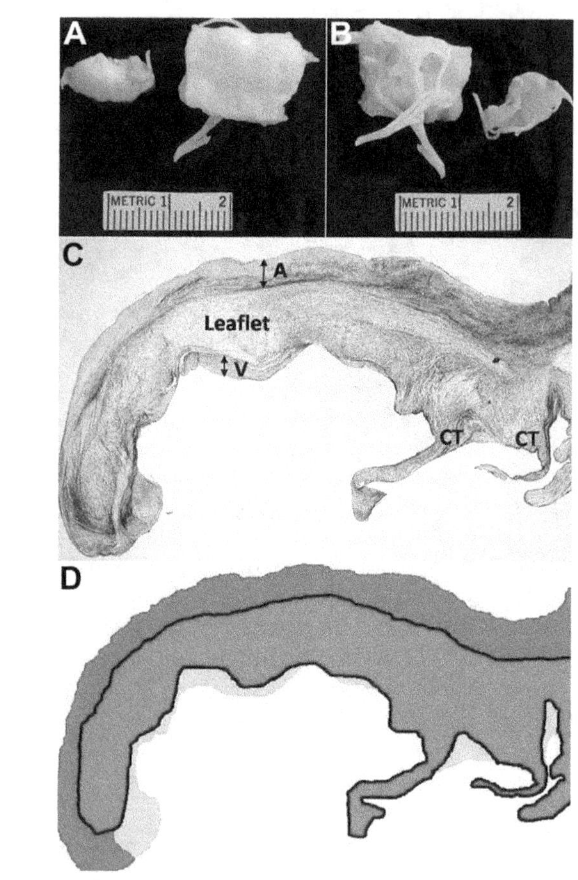

Figure 2   Patient #1 in Table 2

Photographs of the atrial (A) surface **(A)** and ventricular (V) surface **(B)** of a portion of excised posterior mitral valve leaflet. Most chordae are missing from the V surface shown in **B**. **(C)** Photomicrograph showing superimposed fibrous tissue on both the A and V surfaces and increased spongiosa element within the leaflet itself outlined by its black-staining elastic membrane (elastic van Geison, 20×). **(D)** Rendering of the same valve with **red** representing the leaflet itself, **green** representing the superimposed fibrous tissue on the A surface, and **yellow** representing the superimposed fibrous tissue on the V surface. CT = chordae tendineae.

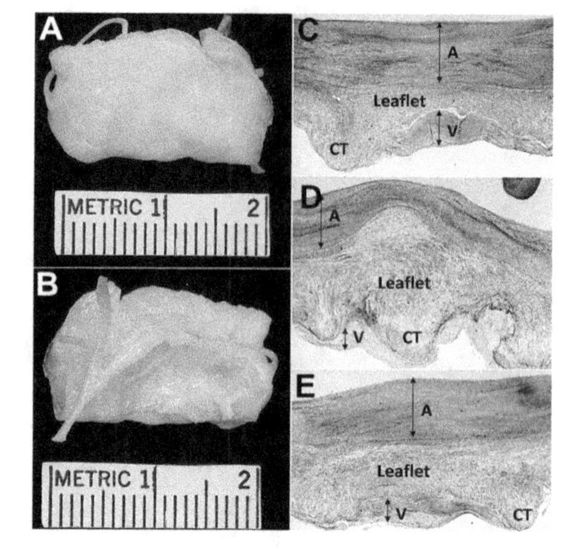

Figure 3   Patient #2 in Table 2

Photographs of the A surface **(A)** and V surface **(B)** of a portion of excised posterior leaflet. Most chordae are missing from the V surface shown in **B**. **(C to E)** Photomicrographs showing superimposed fibrous tissue on both the A and V surfaces and increased spongiosa element within the leaflet itself outlined by its black-staining elastic membrane (elastic van Geison, 40×). Abbreviations as in Figure 2.

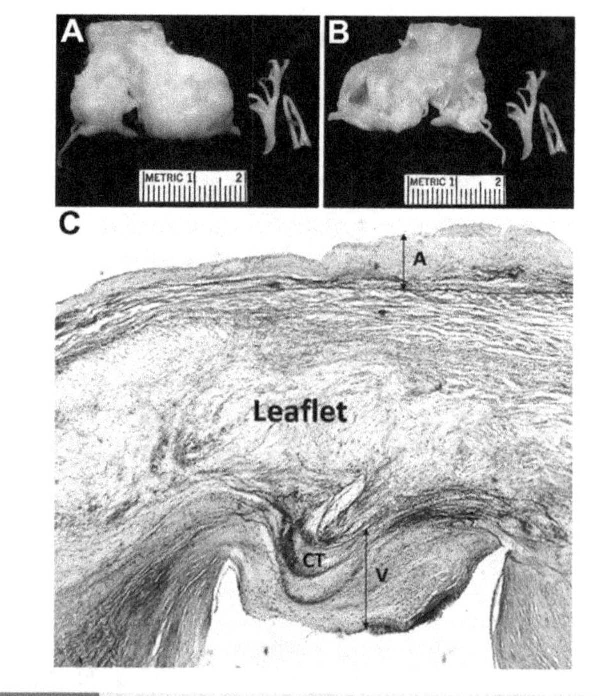

Figure 4   Patient #3 in Table 2

Photographs of the A surface **(A)** and V surface **(B)** of a portion of posterior leaflet. Most chordae are missing from the V surface shown in **B**. **(C)** Photomicrograph showing superimposed fibrous tissue on both the A and V surfaces and severely increased spongiosa element within the leaflet itself outlined by its black-staining elastic membrane (elastic van Geison, 40×). Abbreviations as in Figure 2.

The superimposed fibrous tissue on the atrial and ventricular aspects of the posterior mitral leaflet is quite different histologically. On the atrial aspect, the surface is usually smooth, and the fibrous tissue is dense and contains numerous parallel-lying elastic fibers, simulating in a way the media of an elastic artery. By contrast, the superimposed fibrous tissue on the ventricular surface and surrounding the chordae tends to have an irregular surface, the collagen is less dense, and it contains few, if any, elastic fibers. The atrial surfaces, of course, are the ones making abnormal leaflet contact; the ventricular surfaces are receiving the impact of the left ventricular systolic pressure. The reason for the structural difference between the 2 surfaces is unclear.

That the identification of a ruptured chord is infrequent but that covered (by fibrous tissue) chordae are nearly

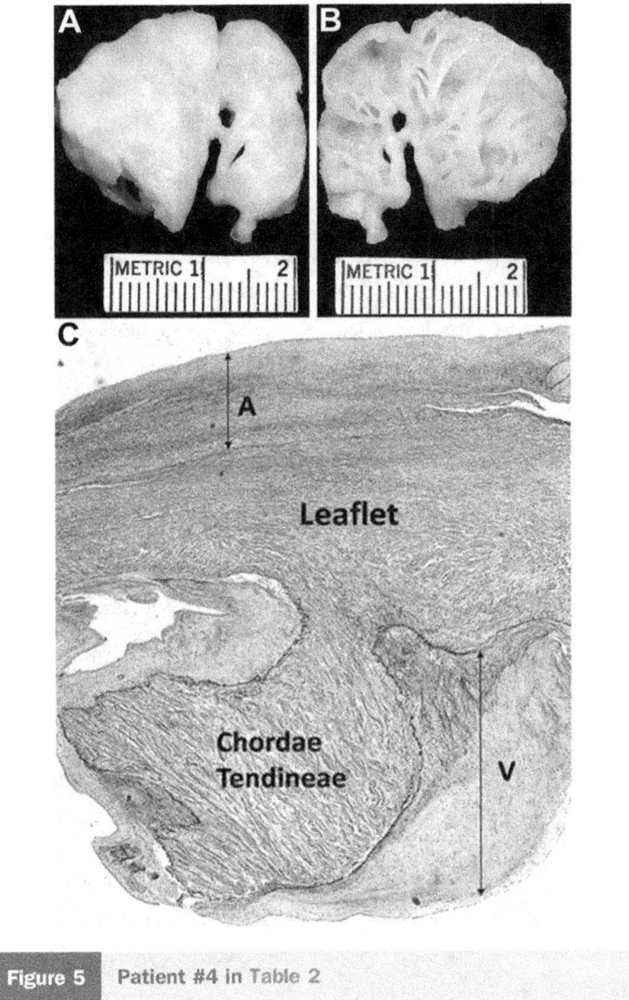

Figure 5   Patient #4 in Table 2

Photographs of the A surface **(A)** and V surface **(B)** of a portion of excised posterior leaflet. Most chordae are missing from or tangled on the V surface shown in **B**. **(C)** Photomicrograph showing superimposed fibrous tissue on both the A and V surfaces and no or minimal increase in the spongiosa element within the leaflet itself, which is outlined by its black-staining elastic membrane (elastic van Geison, 40×). Abbreviations as in Figure 2.

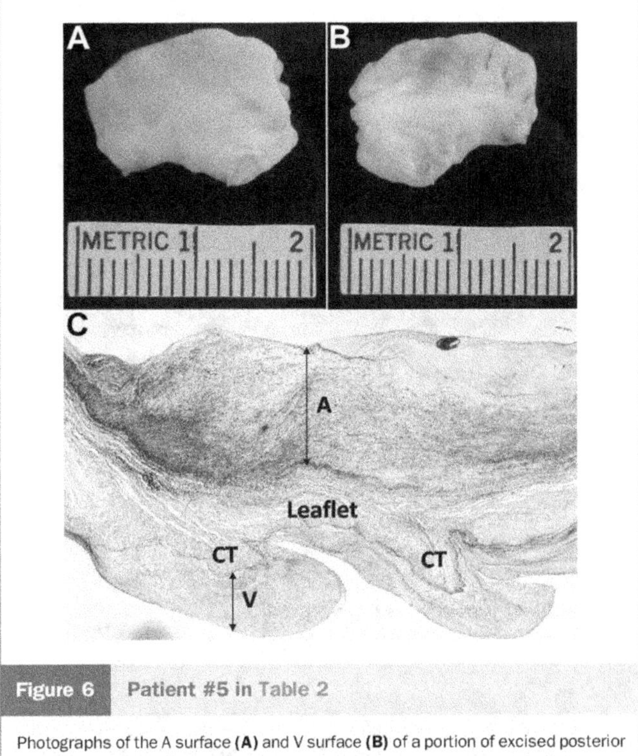

Figure 6   Patient #5 in Table 2

Photographs of the A surface **(A)** and V surface **(B)** of a portion of excised posterior leaflet. All chordae are missing from the V surface shown in **B**. **(C)** Photomicrograph showing superimposed fibrous tissue on both the A and V surfaces and only mildly increased spongiosa element within the leaflet itself, outlined by its black-staining elastic membrane (elastic van Geison, 40×). Abbreviations as in Figure 2.

universal in patients with MVP and MR severe enough to warrant operative repair strongly suggest that most chordal ruptures are clinically silent and occur possibly multiple times through the years. Also, the patients having acute heart failure might have ruptured a primary chord (i.e., one arising from a papillary muscle itself and not one actually attached to the mitral leaflet, as would be the case with a tertiary chord, which would unlikely lead to MR or to a sudden worsening of MR).

This article, of course, follows numerous ones discussing gross and histological features of prolapsed mitral valves examined at either necropsy or after operative excision (1–20). Few, however, mentioned the superimposed fibrous tissue on the leaflet and chordae, probably because elastic-tissue stains were not used, a requirement to see the outline of the underlying leaflet and chordae. Additionally,

none mentioned hidden—previously ruptured—chordae by the overlying fibrous tissue. Thus, chordal rupture in MVP is far more common than previously appreciated (10,13,14,16,21–23).

Elastic-tissue stains were prepared on all histological sections of the operatively excised posterior mitral leaflets, a requirement to separate the superimposed fibrous tissue from the underlying leaflet itself. In all cases, the operative specimen and histological sections of it were studied and described by the same individual (namely, W.C.R.) and not by a variety of persons with varying knowledge of and interest in cardiovascular disease. All patients included had pre-operative echocardiograms described by the reader to be characteristic of MVP. The present report excluded all patients with angiographic evidence of significant coronary narrowing and any patient having coronary artery bypass grafting; all patients with a dysfunctioning aortic valve or aortic valve repair or replacement and all patients with associated mitral stenosis or prior infective endocarditis at any time were also excluded. All these exclusions were an attempt to make certain the patients included herein were a group with "pure" MVP.

Study limitations. We studied only patients with MVP who had MR severe enough to warrant mitral valve repair. Whether our observations hold true for younger patients

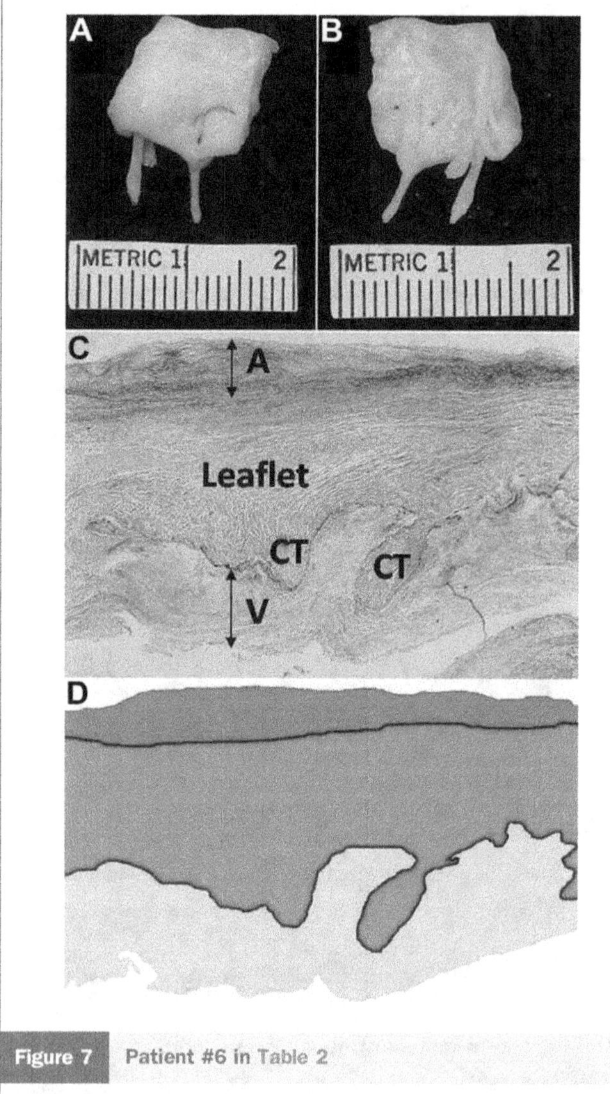

Figure 7 Patient #6 in Table 2

Photographs of the A surface (**A**) and V surface (**B**) of a portion of excised posterior leaflet. Most chordae are missing from the V surface. (**C**) Photomicrograph showing superimposed fibrous tissue on both the A and V surfaces and mildly increased spongiosa element within the leaflet itself, which is outlined by its black-staining elastic membrane (elastic van Geison, 40×). (**D**) Rendering of the same valve with **red** representing the leaflet itself, **green** representing the superimposed fibrous tissue on the A surface, and **yellow** representing the superimposed fibrous tissue on the V surface. Abbreviations as in Figure 2.

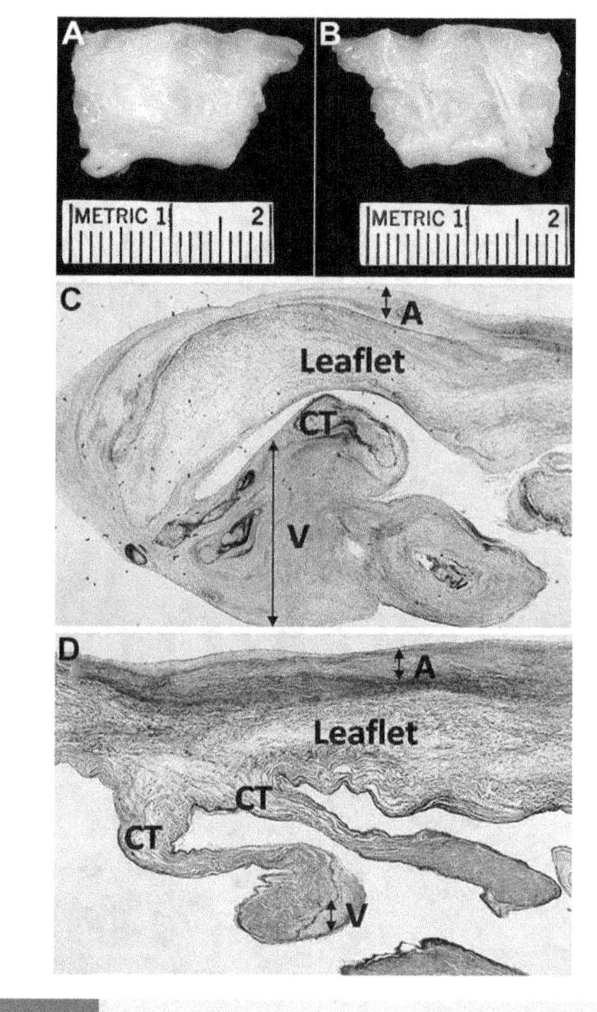

Figure 8 Patient #7 in Table 2

Photographs of the A surface (**A**) and V surface (**B**) of a portion of excised posterior leaflet. Most chordae are missing from the V surface shown in **B**. (**C**) Photomicrograph distally at the free margin showing a large amount of superimposed fibrous tissue on both the A and V surfaces and almost complete replacement of the fibrosa element by the spongiosa element within the leaflet itself outlined by its black-staining elastic membrane (elastic van Geison, 40×). (**D**) Photomicrograph of the same valve to the annulus showing less superimposed fibrous tissue on the A and V surfaces and only a moderate increase in the spongiosa element within the leaflet (elastic van Geison, 40×). Abbreviations as in Figure 2.

(e.g., with mild MR from MVP) is unclear. Additionally, the amount of mitral leaflet tissue available to examine varied from patient to patient. Although all 37 patients had precordial systolic murmurs recorded in the medical record, whether the murmur was pansystolic or late systolic only or accompanied by 1 or more systolic clicks was not recorded. The echocardiograms were interpreted by a number of different echocardiographers. Details of the thickness of the mitral leaflets were not recorded in any echocardiographic report and not by any surgeon at operation.

Conclusions

This study of operatively-excised posterior mitral leaflets in patients with MR secondary to MVP indicates that the leaflet thickening is the result primarily of superimposed fibrous tissue on both surfaces of the leaflet and that previously ruptured chordae, nearly universal, are usually covered by the superimposed fibrous tissue on the ventricular surface by the time of operative intervention.

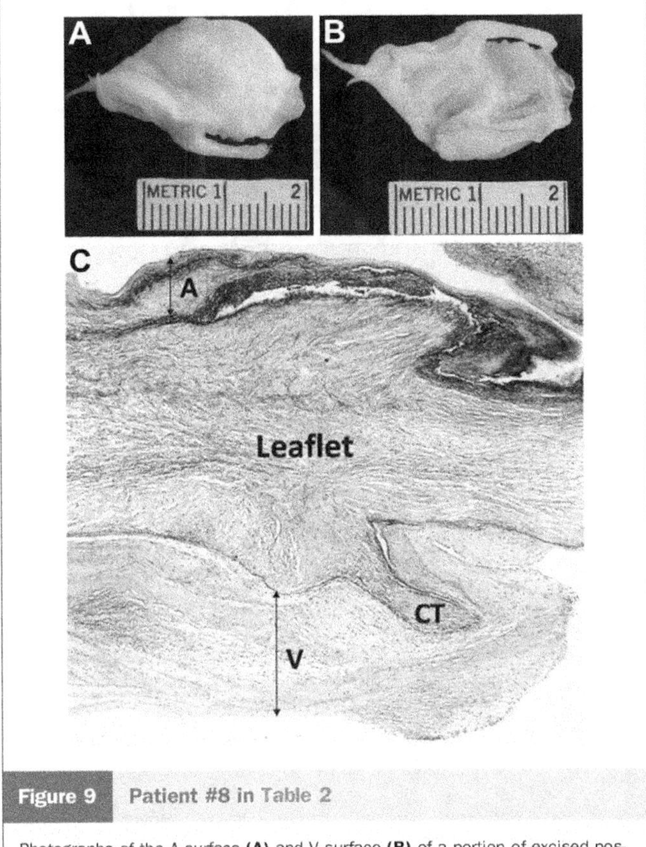

Figure 9 — Patient #8 in Table 2

Photographs of the A surface (A) and V surface (B) of a portion of excised posterior leaflet. Most chordae are missing from the V surface. (C) Photomicrograph showing superimposed fibrous tissue on both the A and V surfaces and increased spongiosa element within the valve leaflet itself, outlined by its black-staining elastic membrane (elastic van Geison, 40×). Abbreviations as in Figure 2.

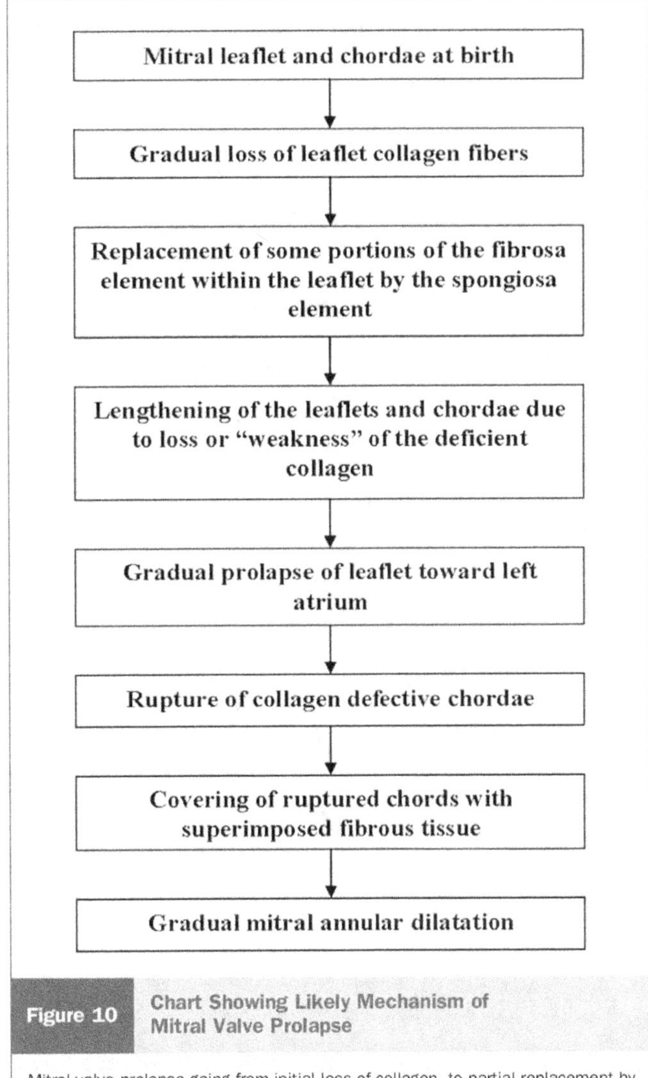

Figure 10 — Chart Showing Likely Mechanism of Mitral Valve Prolapse

Mitral valve prolapse going from initial loss of collagen, to partial replacement by the spongiosa element, to leaflet elongation and chordal rupture with focal leaflet prolapse, and gradual thickening due to superimposed fibrous tissue.

Table 2 — Comparison of Various Variables Among 8 Patients Having Isolated MV Repair for MV Prolapse Whose Valves Are Illustrated Both Grossly and Histologically

Patient #	Figure #	Age (yrs)	Sex	Race	Pressures (mm Hg)			EF (%)	MV Weight (g)
					RV (s/d)	LV (s/d)	Aorta (s/d)		
1	2	43	M	W	34/15	112/12	111/74	70	1.02
2	3	46	F	W	26/10	101/13	104/55	40	0.64
3	4	48	M	W	38/14	102/23	106/67	65	1.94
4	5	54	M	W	31/11	—	120/55*	65	1.61
5	6	54	F	W	—	—	100/55*	—	0.33
6	7	55	M	W	34/10	137/19	135/80	70	0.31
7	8	59	M	A	41/9	116/14	121/85	30	0.47
8	9	66	M	W	16/2	92/6	96/69	—	0.81

*Indirect blood pressure measurement.

s/d = systole/diastole; other abbreviations as in Table 1.

Reprint requests and correspondence: Dr. William C. Roberts, Baylor Heart and Vascular Institute, Baylor University Medical Center at Dallas, 3500 Gaston Avenue, Dallas, Texas 75246. E-mail: wc.roberts@baylorhealth.edu.

REFERENCES

1. Fernex M, Fernex C. Mucoid degenerescence of the mitral valve; functional repercussions. Helv Med Acta 1958;25:694–705.
2. Read RC, Thal AP, Wendt VE. Symptomatic valvular myxomatous transformation (the floppy valve syndrome). A possible forme frusta of the Marfan syndrome. Circulation 1965;32:897–910.
3. Bittar N, Sosa JA. The billowing mitral valve leaflet. Report on fourteen patients. Circulation 1968;38:763–70.
4. Trent JK, Adelman AG, Wigle ED, Silver MD. Morphology of a prolapsed posterior mitral valve leaflet. Am Heart J 1970;79:539–43.
5. McCarthy LJ, Wolf PL. Mucoid degeneration of heart valves: "blue valve syndrome". Am J Clin Pathol 1970;54:852–6.
6. Shappell SD, Marshall CE. Ballooning posterior leaflet syndrome. Syncope and sudden death. Arch Intern Med 1975;135:664–7.
7. Davies MJ, Moore BP, Braimbridge MV. The floppy mitral valve. Study of incidence, pathology, and complications in surgical, necropsy, and forensic material. Br Heart J 1978;40:468–81.
8. Olsen EGJ, Al-Rufaie HK. The floppy mitral valve. Study on pathogenesis. Br Heart J 1980;44:674–83.
9. Rippe J, Fishbein MC, Carabello B, et al. Primary myxomatous degeneration of cardiac valves. Clinical, pathological, haemodynamic, and echocardiographic profile. Br Heart J 1980;44:621–9.
10. Hickey AJ, Wilcken DEL, Wright JS, Warren BS. Primary (spontaneous) chordal rupture: relation to myxomatous valve disease and mitral valve prolapse. J Am Coll Cardiol 1985;5:1341–6.
11. van der Bel-Kahn J, Duren DR, Becker AE. Isolated mitral valve prolapse: chordal architecture as an anatomic basis in older patients. J Am Coll Cardiol 1985;5:1335–40.
12. Hanson TP, Edwards BS, Edwards JE. Pathology of surgically excised mitral valves. Arch Pathol Lab Med 1985;109:823–8.
13. Olson LJ, Subramanian R, Ackermann DM, Orszulak TA, Edwards WD. Surgical pathology of the mitral valve: a study of 712 cases spanning 21 years. Mayo Clin Proc 1987;62:22–34.
14. Roberts WC, McIntosh CL, Wallace RB. Mechanisms of severe mitral regurgitation in mitral valve prolapse determined from analysis of operatively excised valves. Am Heart J 1987;113:1316–23.
15. Virmani R, Atkinson JB, Forman MB. The pathology of mitral valve prolapse. Herz 1988;13:215–26.
16. Turri M, Thiene G, Bortolotti U, Mazzucco A, Gallucci V. Surgical pathology of disease of the mitral valve, with special reference to lesions promoting valvular incompetence. Int J Cardiol 1989;22:213–9.
17. Dollar AL, Roberts WC. Morphologic comparison of patients with mitral valve prolapse who died suddenly with patients who died from severe valvular dysfunction or other conditions. J Am Coll Cardiol 1991;17:921–31.
18. Agozzino L, Falco A, de Vivo F, de Vinventiis C, de Luca L, Esposito S, Cotrufo M. Surgical pathology of the mitral valve: gross and histological study of 1288 surgically excised valves. Int J Cardiol 1992;37:79–89.
19. Shirani J, Roberts WC. Clinical and morphologic features of mitral valve prolapse in octogenarians. Am J Cardiol 1993;72:1316–9.
20. Butany J, Privitera S, David TE. Mitral valve prolapse: an atypical variation of the anatomy. Can J Cardiol 2003;19:1367–73.
21. Cooley DA, Gerami S, Hallman GL, Wukasch DC, Hall RJ. Mitral insufficiency due to myxomatous transformation: "floppy valve syndrome". J Cardiovasc Surg 1972;13:346–9.
22. Chadraratna PA, Aronow WS. Incidence of ruptured chordae tendineae in mitral valve prolapse syndrome. An echocardiographic study. Chest 1979;75:334–9.
23. Grenadier E, Alpan G, Keidar S, Palant A. The prevalence of ruptured chordae tendineae in the mitral valve prolapse syndrome. Am Heart J 1983;105:603–10.

Key Words: mitral regurgitation ▪ mitral valve prolapse ▪ mitral valve repair.